Interventions for Schizophrenia

Emma Williams

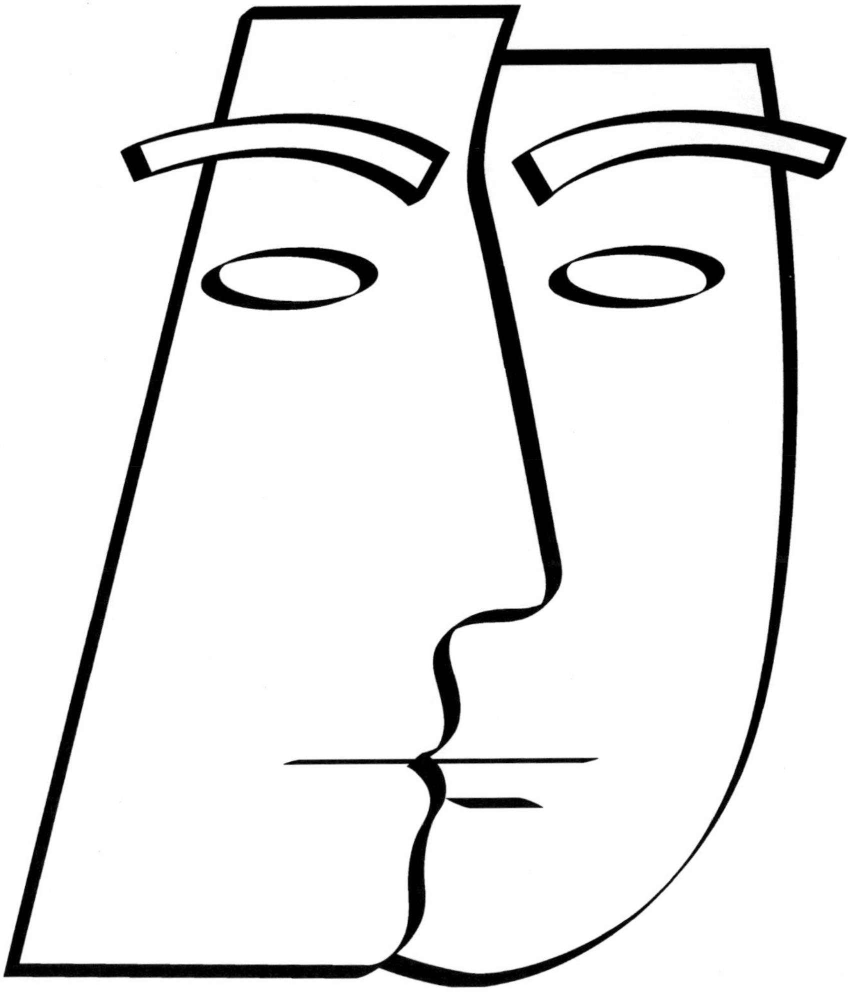

Interventions for Schizophrenia

Emma Williams

Speechmark

Speechmark Publishing Ltd · Telford Road · Bicester · Oxon OX26 4LQ · UK

Dedication

To Loris
Our steps will always rhyme.

Acknowledgement

I would like to thank the many enthusiastic and dedicated colleagues that I have been so fortunate to work with at the Wallingford Clinic and the Oxford Clinic. Particular thanks to Patsy Holly, Rebecca Kelly and Gavin Garman.

Special thanks to Krissi Hartley-Morris for her expert skills in preparing the manuscript, meeting impossible deadlines and for being such a wonderful person.

First published in 2004 by
Speechmark Publishing Ltd, Telford Road, Bicester, Oxon OX26 4LQ, UK
Tel: +44 (0) 1869 244 644 Fax: +44 (0) 1869 320 040
www.speechmark.net

002-5137/Printed in the United Kingdom/1010

British Library Cataloguing in Publication Data
Williams, Emma
Interventions for schizophrenia
1. Schizophrenia — Treatment 2. Schizophrenia
I. Title
616.8′9806

ISBN 0 86388 435 0
ISBN 978 0 86388 4351

Contents

Handouts and Worksheets

MODULE 1

Handouts

Worksheets

MODULE 2

Handouts

Worksheets

MODULE 3

Handouts

Worksheets

MODULE 4

Handouts

Worksheets

MODULE 5

Handouts

Worksheets

Figures, Table and Boxes

Figures

Table

Boxes

Psychological Interventions for Schizophrenia: Theory & Practice

PART I

Philosophy of approach

The philosophy of this approach sets the context for the interventions. The programme has three underlying tenets: the importance of the therapeutic alliance, responsivity of interventions and addressing multiple needs.

Establishing a positive therapeutic alliance is vital in enabling clients to engage with treatment; this is one of the primary tasks of the therapist. The therapeutic relationship is the core ingredient in helping people with a diagnosis of schizophrenia. It is known that 30 per cent of the treatment effect of therapy is common to all types of psychological therapy, whereas only 15 per cent of the effect is related to the specific psychological treatment offered. The common factor appears to be the formation of a collaborative, supportive and non-judgemental relationship. Respect and understanding help people to get better! The National Institute for Clinical Excellence (NICE) recognises the importance of working in partnership with service users 'in an atmosphere of hope and optimism' (NICE 2002).

The responsivity principle highlights that interventions must be sensitive and tailored to the client's abilities and capabilities. Clients have different levels of cognitive and intellectual functioning as well as different interpersonal and learning styles. The programme should be delivered in a way that is compatible with the needs and abilities of the client. Therapy goals should not be pre-set and prescriptive, but decided collaboratively.

Clients have multiple needs and require a comprehensive approach that can target specific needs, for example psychological, clinical, social, occupational. Promotion of recovery is a primary aim and interventions such as cognitive-behavioural therapy to prevent relapse and reduce symptoms must be set in the context of the strengths and needs of the client.

An integrated approach

The programme draws together the major psychological contributions to the management and treatment of schizophrenia over the past 20 years. This comprehensive approach can be used by a variety of mental health professionals in a variety of settings.

The British Psychological Society's major report *Recent Advances in Understanding Mental Illness and Psychotic Experiences*' (British Psychological Society, 2000) states that despite the effectiveness and popularity of psychological treatments they are not yet widely provided by the National Health Service for people who have psychotic experiences. The report concludes that 'psychological help should be available to every service user who wants it, either individually or in a group, depending on their preference. This is one of the most important messages of this report.' They further conclude that 'all mental health workers should be able to use psychological frameworks of understanding in their work with service users'.

This manual brings together a variety of specific interventions known to be effective in the management of schizophrenia in order to provide a broad-based and effective intervention programme. A variety of techniques commonly used in the treatment of mental health problems has been modified to apply specifically to the problems encountered by people with a diagnosis of schizophrenia. They include interventions such as symptom management, cognitive behavioural therapy, coping skill enhancement, social skills training and relapse prevention strategies.

While psychodynamic and psychoanalytically oriented approaches do not directly inform this approach, they are influential in emphasising the importance of the process as well as the content of therapy, and in highlighting the importance of concepts such as 'unconscious deception' or the defensive role of some psychotic experiences as well as the importance of underlying conflicts such as grief and loss.

The psychological intervention programme has a cognitive behavioural framework and uses the vulnerability stress model as its primary theoretical underpinning.

The 'schizophrenias'

Within the range of severe mental illness the diagnosis of schizophrenia is the most common. Approximately one person in 100 will be diagnosed with schizophrenia during their lifetime (Birchwood et al, 1988). The prevalence of schizophrenia is estimated to be between 0.2 per cent and 1 per cent; this means that in Britain between 100,000 and 500,000 people will be diagnosed with schizophrenia at any one time (Torrey, 1987). Approximately 70 per cent of all psychiatric inpatients have a diagnosis of schizophrenia.

Schizophrenia is one of the 'psychotic' disorders; that is, those disorders that are characterised by the symptoms of delusions and hallucinations. Other psychotic disorders include schizoaffective disorder, delusional disorder, brief psychotic disorder, psychotic disorder due to a general medical condition and substance-induced psychotic disorder. Schizophrenia itself is further subdivided into five types: paranoid, disorganised, catatonic, undifferentiated and residual (American Psychiatric Association, DSM IV-TR, 2000).

That there is such a range of diverse and overlapping diagnoses indicates that the disorders are not easily defined or differentiated. Indeed, reviewing notes of people with a long history of contact with psychiatric services often reveals a list of previous diagnoses including various types of schizophrenia and different psychotic disorders, as well as other disorders such as personality disorder and other mental health problems. Some mental health professionals believe that the specific categorisation of different mental illnesses should be abolished in favour of general categories such as psychosis and neurosis, with treatment, including medication, being prescribed to target specific symptoms rather than informed by a specific diagnosis.

While it is recognised that a diagnosis of schizophrenia has significant overlap with other psychotic disorders such as major depression, bipolar affective disorder and persistent delusional states, it is distinctive enough in terms of its onset, course and prognosis to remain a helpful concept in attempting to understand the variety of problems associated with schizophrenia.

People with a diagnosis of schizophrenia tend to experience symptoms within two general categories: positive and negative symptoms. Positive symptoms are those which are additional, or excessive, to normal functioning. Primarily *delusions*: persecutory, religious, referential; *hallucinations*: visual, auditory, tactile, olfactory; *unusual speech*: derailment, tangential; *unusual behaviour*: agitation, dysinhibition.

Negative symptoms are those which reflect a loss or diminution of normal functioning, such as reduction in emotional expression, reduction of fluency in thought and speech, loss of volition.

Each person's experience of the disorder is unique, and is influenced by their personal, family and social histories. In addition to the nature of the disorder, the outcome, course and response to treatment also vary widely. Having such experiences is frequently distressing, interferes substantially with the ability to enjoy a 'normal' life and alienates the person from others. People with a diagnosis of schizophrenia often experience not only the problems of the illness itself, but also the stigma, social ostracism and prejudice associated with mental illness. In addition the experience of the psychiatric system itself can be traumatic and can include loss of rights, compulsory treatment and loss of liberty.

Psychological models of schizophrenia

Medically informed models tend to use a disease concept of schizophrenia. The illness is viewed as entirely separate from the normal healthy 'not ill' state. Medical researchers are primarily concerned with identifying the cause of such an illness and focus on possible biochemical, genetic, anatomical or other biological abnormalities. Psychiatric treatments are primarily physical with antipsychotic medication being the primary, and frequently the only, treatment intervention offered.

Psychological models have tended to view the disorder as on a continuum from normality to dysfunction, and attempt to examine predisposing vulnerability and protective factors, as well as taking into consideration the cognitive and emotional underpinnings of the disorder.

While medical and psychological models view the concept of schizophrenia differently, they are not mutually exclusive, and indeed all psychological processes are associated with specific biological responses and brain activity. In terms of the potential causes of schizophrenia, it is likely that there are specific interactions between psychological, sociological and biological factors. As with most complex problems the answer is usually multifactorial!

Several psychological models of schizophrenia have been postulated. Claridge (1990) describes a dimensional model of schizophrenia in which the disorder is hypothesised to arise from an interaction between the underlying disposition and a range of developmental and triggering factors.

Bentall (1990) proposed that the concept of schizophrenia should be abandoned and replaced with a focus on individual symptoms such as auditory hallucinations. Proponents of this approach examine symptoms using models from cognitive psychology, such as perception and language.

The most widely used psychological model of schizophrenia is the vulnerability stress model (Zubin and Spring, 1977). The original vulnerability stress model proposed that individuals are made vulnerable to developing schizophrenia by their genetic composition and acquired traits. This vulnerability is mediated by coping ability, social competence and coping effort. External stressors such as adverse life events can disable coping responses, and episodes of psychiatric illness can then develop in such individuals.

There have been several revisions of the original model, which have expanded the framework to include a variety of protecting and potentiating factors (eg Neuchterlein, 1987). The expanded model is presented in Figure 1.

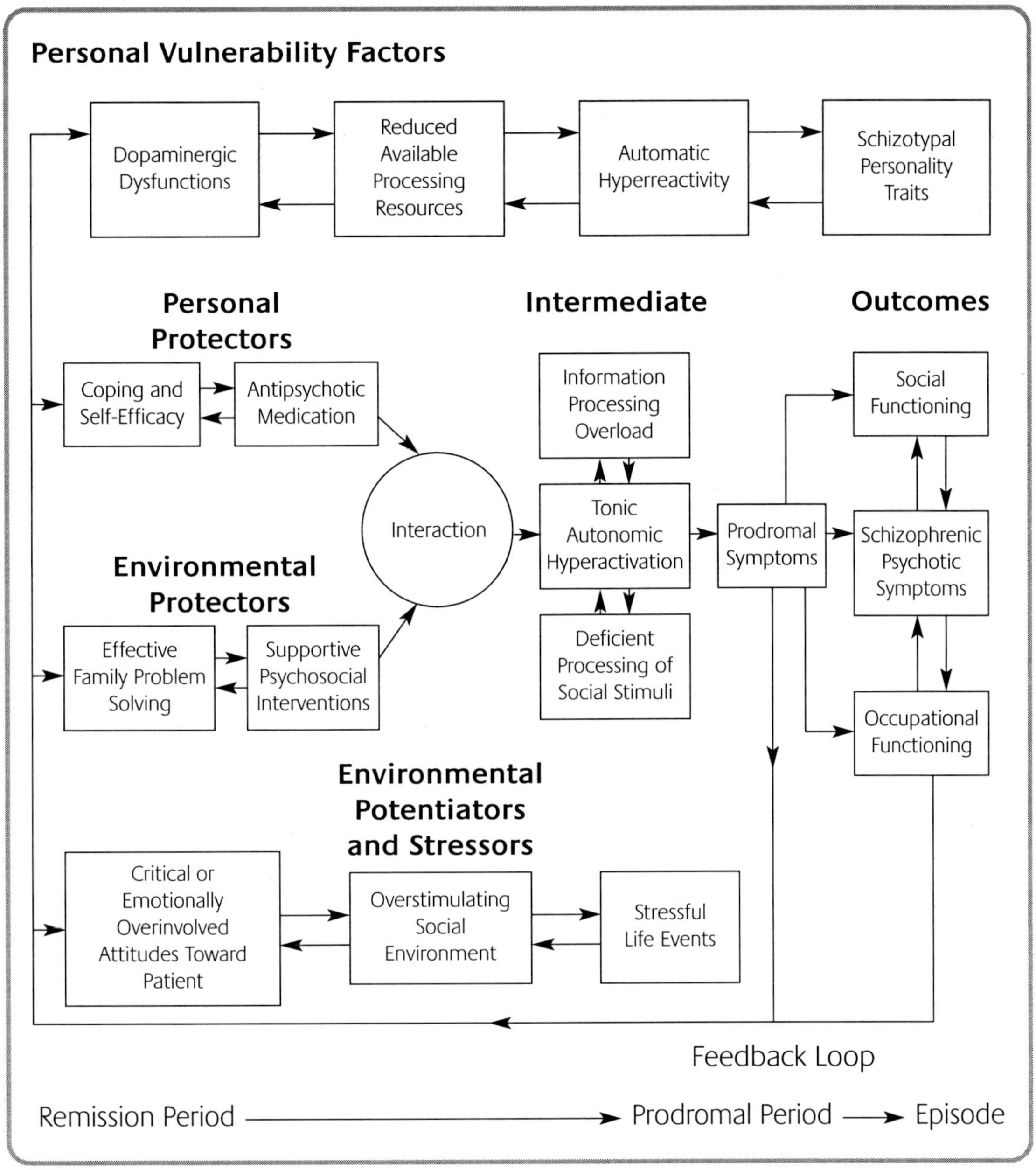

Figure 1 Heuristic conceptual framework for possible factors in the development of schizophrenic episodes
Source: Neuchterlein (1987), with permission (© Springer Verlag).

Personal vulnerability factors include neurobiological abnormalities such as dopamine levels, neurophysiological deficits such as selective attention difficulties, electrodermal overactivity which can lead to hyperresponsivity, and personality traits present since early childhood which might lead to social interaction difficulties.

Personal protective factors include the person's coping abilities and self-efficacy, that is, their potential to manage stress effectively and to overcome adverse circumstances. The model proposes that antipsychotic medication is also a protecting factor which might, for example, reduce the effect of any neurotransmitter abnormality and thereby minimise the effect of personal vulnerability.

Environmental potentiators and stressors play an important part as these can precipitate psychotic episodes in vulnerable people. The more vulnerable the person is the less external stress is required to trigger such an episode. Potentiating factors can include critical or emotionally laden attitudes, commonly known as 'expressed emotion' in close relationships, such as with parents, spouse, carers. Overstimulating social environments and stressful life events are frequently contributing factors.

Environmental protectors are those factors which improve the person's ability to withstand adverse circumstances and therefore increase their tolerance to stress thresholds. These include effective family functioning, such as the ability to problem solve, as well as health and social circumstances which might be the target of specific psychosocial interventions.

Intermediate states such as information processing problems, autonomic nervous system problems and social communication problems are seen as contributing to the emergence of prodromal symptoms. These factors can therefore be seen as early warning signs to an episode of psychosis. However, the model proposes that such a relapse can be averted by increasing the protectors or reducing the sources of external stress.

The outcome therefore depends on a number of factors. This provides a therapeutically optimistic model, which does not view psychotic relapse as inevitable but suggests that interventions at many different points might influence the system to reduce the risk of a psychotic episode.

The use and effectiveness of psychological treatments

> 'Psychological treatments should be an indispensable part of the treatment options available for service users and their families in the effort to promote recovery. Those with the best evidence of effectiveness are cognitive behavioural therapy and family interventions. These should be used to prevent relapse, to reduce symptoms, increase insight and promote adherence to medication.'
>
> *National Institute for Clinical Excellence*
> *Schizophrenia Guideline, 2002.*

The development of psychological treatment approaches to help people with a diagnosis of schizophrenia has primarily been driven by three factors. The first factor is the limitations of the medical model of diagnosis and treatment of symptoms by medication. The alleviation of symptoms of schizophrenia addresses only a small proportion of the difficulties and experiences of people with such a diagnosis. Psychological models have widened the focus of treatment to include the role of life events, stress, family and other interpersonal relationships as well as the person's social and psychological histories.

Second, while antipsychotic medication has greatly improved the lives of many there are a substantial number of people whose symptoms are 'medication resistant' or who respond only partially to such treatment. Full remission of psychotic symptoms is found in less than two-thirds of people with a diagnosis of schizophrenia (Shepherd et al, 1989). In a community sample of outpatients receiving long-term depot medication, 23 per cent continued to experience residual psychotic symptoms (Curson et al, 1985), while in a long-stay psychiatric hospital population, the figure was almost half (Curson et al, 1988). People experiencing symptoms such as continuing hallucinations or delusions have been found not only to be more likely to need continued hospitalisation but also to find such experiences very distressing; the content of the majority of voices is abusive and denigratory (Nyani and David, 1996). More than 25 per cent of people with a diagnosis of schizophrenia have made a serious suicide attempt in response to auditory hallucinations (Falloon and Talbot, 1981). Antipsychotic medication, while effective in many cases, can also produce a range of unpleasant and distressing side effects. Often, compliance to prescribed medication is limited due to side effects and other factors, and therefore the potential effectiveness of medication is reduced because people do not adhere to the prescribed regime. Psychological approaches have challenged the traditional views of psychotic symptoms as either amenable or not amendable to treatment by medication, by developing ways that the person themself can cope with, challenge and control such experiences. Psychological approaches can also promote adherence to medication.

Third, the growth and organisation of user and carer involvement in mental health services has led to a call for a more collaborative and client-centred approach to treatment. Whereas medical treatments are often prescriptive and directed without the full involvement of the patients, psychological approaches are based on reaching a formulation of the person's difficulties by the development of a collaborative, therapeutic relationship.

There are several psychological approaches which focus on different aspects of helping people with a diagnosis of schizophrenia. Interventions include family intervention programmes, social skills training and management and modification of specific symptoms. Evidence of the effectiveness for six common psychological interventions is reviewed below.

Social skills training

The aim of social skills approaches is to improve psychosocial functioning. The focus is on the practical use of important interpersonal skills such as problem solving, assertiveness and communication skills. Such approaches have been described as examining and improving deficits in a person's receiving, processing and sending skills (Vaccaro and Roberts, 1992). People with a diagnosis of schizophrenia might have problems with attention and concentration, as well as positive symptoms which interfere with the reception of social information. Processing such information can also be adversely affected by difficulties in generating, evaluating and selecting a response. Sending skills can be disrupted by disorganised speech and thought processes, as well as verbal and non-verbal communication deficits. Most social skills training uses modelling, rehearsal and behavioural practice in order to improve social functioning.

Social skills training has been found to significantly increase knowledge and skill levels in people with a diagnosis of schizophrenia (Wallace and Liberman, 1985). There is also some evidence that social skills training can extend to the prevention, or at least the delay, of relapse, with some researchers suggesting as much as a halving of relapse rates when social skills training techniques are combined with medication (Hogarty, 1984). However, reviewers of social skills training research have found that although such training can lead to improvements in role play tests, these commonly fail to be maintained over time, and often fail to generalise to community settings (Emmelkamp, 1994).

A meta-analytic review of 23 studies of social skills training with inpatients with a diagnosis of schizophrenia found that role-play-based measures showed greater improvement than did naturalistic measures. Self-rated assertiveness showed some improvement, however no significant differences were found in general functioning, symptomatology or discharge and relapse rates (Benton and Schroeder, 1990).

It is generally concluded that there is some evidence for the effectiveness of social skills training, although generalisation remains problematic. Improving interpersonal skills such as problem solving, communication, assertiveness and interpersonal confidence is an essential component of the current programme. Opportunity to practise and rehearse such skills in order for them to become internalised and therefore to generalise to other settings is vital. Ensuring that the skills taught are those which the person sees as valuable and meaningful will aid this process.

Family intervention programmes

The development of family intervention programmes was largely a response to findings in the 1970s that the quality of the family relationship could predict relapse in people with a diagnosis of schizophrenia (Brown et al, 1972; Vaughn and Leff, 1976). It was found that relapse rates were significantly higher in those people who lived with relatives who were excessively critical, and/or overinvolved. 'Expressed emotion', as this concept is described, is not seen as causing schizophrenia, but as a contributory factor in relapse. Expressed emotion has also been found to be related to the difficulties of caring for relatives with a diagnosis of schizophrenia.

Family intervention programmes aim to reduce the risk of relapse by improving family functioning. The programmes tend to focus on acknowledging and examining the 'burden of care,' building on the positive areas of family functioning, improving family cohesiveness and stability. Techniques from systemic psychotherapy are used, together with cognitive behavioural therapy approaches. Specific interventions can include goal setting, problem solving, cognitive restructuring and stress reduction techniques. Such programmes are predominantly conducted in the community when the person with the diagnosis of schizophrenia is living at home.

A review of family intervention programmes found significant reductions in relapse rates. At approximately one year, rates in treated families varied from 6 per cent to 23 per cent, whereas those in a non-treatment comparison group relapsed at between 40 per cent and 53 per cent. Levels of expressed emotion were found to be reduced by intervention, and generally household, social and employment functioning improved compared with the no intervention control group. At two years the differences in relapse were less marked but still significant, suggesting that intervention delays, but does not ultimately prevent, relapse (Lam, 1991). The family intervention programme, which continued contact over the two-year follow up period, obtained the lowest relapse rates suggesting that maintenance models of continuing care are likely to be the most beneficial (Falloon et al, 1982). Expressed emotion is also an important factor when the carers are mental health staff. It has been found that up to 40 per cent of staff demonstrate high levels of expressed emotion, mainly criticism (Kuipers and Moore, 1995).

A systematic review of psychological interventions for schizophrenia concluded that family interventions aimed at enhancing family structure and encouraging positive social interactions can lead to a decreased relapse rate for one to two years by a factor of two to three (Roth and Fonagy, 1996).

Family intervention approaches emphasise the importance of acknowledging the wider context in which the person lives, and how this can impact on their progress. General cognitive behavioural techniques, such as cognitive restructuring and stress reduction, can be used, together with enhancing positive areas of functioning. Expressed emotion research, while primarily concerned with the interpersonal functioning within families, can equally be applied to mental health professionals as carers, particularly in an inpatient setting. The current programme focuses on forming collaborative therapeutic relationships with clients in order to reduce the impact of this potentially powerful environmental potentiator of relapse. Family intervention work is also drawn on in order to help examine the person's interpersonal relationships and to suggest strategies for improving relationships.

Behavioural interventions

Behavioural interventions aimed at reducing the impact of positive symptoms, most commonly auditory hallucinations, have included a variety of strategies such as relaxation, distraction, use of ear plugs, exercise, focusing, thought stopping, systematic desensitisation and exposure.

A review of psychological interventions for auditory hallucinations concluded that there was insufficient evidence to favour any one technique. Almost all the strategies produced some benefit to some patients (Shergill et al, 1998). Reduction in psychological distress associated with auditory hallucinations and increased feelings of control over the experience of such symptoms are commonly the target of such interventions rather than the elimination of symptoms. Focusing techniques which emphasise self-monitoring, and paying attention to the hallucinations, have been found to decrease the duration of associated distress (Bentall et al, 1994). This might be due to the person directing attention to documenting symptoms and thereby distancing themselves from the subjective experience. It has also been proposed that such interventions may desensitise people to their auditory hallucinations, and therefore act in a similar way to behavioural strategies which concentrate on reducing associated anxiety through relaxation and thought stopping techniques (Shergill et al, 1998).

Distraction techniques appear to be most successful if meaningful competing auditory stimulation is used. Auditory stimulation has been found to reduce the frequency of auditory hallucinations (Margo et al, 1981).

Within the current programme, behavioural techniques such as attentional switching, distraction, focusing and relaxation techniques are encouraged and coping strategy enhancement described. In addition behavioural experiments which allow people to test out whether their thoughts and beliefs are in fact accurate representations of their experience in the real world are also very helpful in examining psychotic experiences.

Cognitive therapy: CT

Cognitive approaches are based on the premiss that psychological difficulties depend on how people think about or interpret events, how they respond to these events and how it makes them feel. Cognitive therapy (CT) aims to help the person to examine their thoughts, feelings and behaviours, and to recognise unhelpful thinking patterns and behaviours in order to modify them to improve their psychological health.

Cognitive behavioural approaches have been used successfully in the treatment of depression, anxiety, obsessional problems, phobias, anger and personality disorders. They have also been applied to the treatment of hallucinations and delusions.

The potential usefulness of cognitive therapy for auditory hallucinations is suggested by several findings. For example, some people who hear voices have difficulty in distinguishing their own thoughts from voices with an external origin (Morrison and Haddock, 1997). It has also been found that hallucinations can be exacerbated by high levels of emotional arousal (Margo et al, 1981). In addition, people's beliefs and explanations about their voices affect their subjective distress (Chadwick and Birchwood, 1994). CT for auditory hallucinations therefore focuses on gaining an understanding of the nature, content and role of the voices, reducing stress or arousal, examining beliefs associated with hallucinations, and examining and if necessary modifying thoughts, feelings and behaviours associated with the hallucinations.

A controlled trial of CT with 20 patients and 20 matched controls, where the treatment comprised individual and group CT focusing on challenging key beliefs, examining inconsistencies in explanations of symptoms and developing coping strategies, found significant improvements in the treatment group. The treatment group was also discharged from hospital sooner and had significantly fewer residual symptoms at nine-month follow up (Drury et al, 1996).

CT for psychotic symptoms is a relatively recent treatment; however, two comprehensive reviews have concluded that CT for auditory hallucinations is indeed effective (Haddock et al, 1998; Shergill et al, 1998).

CT for delusional beliefs has developed from the work of cognitive therapists such as Aaron Beck on the modification of thoughts and beliefs associated with depression and other emotional disorders. Delusions had been viewed as so bizarre and beyond reason that they could not be modified or changed by psychological means, however if delusions are viewed as on a continuum with normal beliefs, over-valued ideas and prejudices, this suggests more optimism in the ability to change such beliefs. Delusional beliefs, like prejudices, are firmly held, resistant to change and reinforced by selective attention. However, there is evidence that delusional beliefs, while not usually open to direct challenge, can be modified by discussing with the person the possible alternative explanations, examining and testing out supporting evidence for the belief. CT has been found to be of benefit in reducing the level of conviction in delusions, as well as the interference they cause and associated distress (Chadwick and Lowe, 1994). A 25 per cent reduction in symptom severity measured by standard psychiatric rating scales has also been found in a large randomised control trial of CT for psychosis, with reduction in delusional beliefs being particularly successful (Kuipers et al, 1997).

In summary, the ability to gain some control over distressing symptoms such as hallucinations and delusions, to reduce the strength or frequency of such symptoms, and even to eliminate them altogether, has been achieved by cognitive interventions. The use of these approaches is a major part of this programme.

Early intervention

Early intervention programmes are based on the premiss that the earlier in the development of psychosis a person is diagnosed and treated, the better the long-term outcome. Early intervention involves identifying the early warning signs to a potential psychotic episode, and offering help as soon as possible. Suitable clients for this approach are considered to be those with a history of repeated relapse, or those who are deemed to be at high risk of relapse: for example those with a history of medication non-adherence, on low doses of medication, living alone or in high expressed emotion environments. It is generally viewed as counterindicated with clients experiencing ongoing residual psychotic symptoms as it is hard to discriminate a prodrome from existing symptoms (Birchwood et al, 1992).

Early intervention generally involves engagement and education, which emphasises the importance of recognising prodromes and potential relapse in order to initiate treatment. It also involves gaining detailed information about the individual's prodromal signs or 'relapse signature', monitoring of potential relapse signs and ensuring the availability of a rapid response such as access to mental health professionals, counselling and medication. Studies of people experiencing their first episode of acute psychosis indicate that early intervention before or during this period produces significantly positive effects over the course of the illness. One study followed up 253 first episode clients over two years, of whom 120 were a control group. The period of time between the individual's loss of well-being and presentation to services – the 'duration of untreated illness' – was found to be predictive of likelihood of relapse (MacMillan et al, 1986).

Early intervention programmes focus on relapse, and demonstrate that early recognition of relapse signs followed by timely and appropriate responses can reduce the impact or even prevent relapse, as well as improve long-term outcome. The focus on self-monitoring and the ability to notice and predict potential relapse is a key component of the current programme.

Relapse prevention

Several of the concepts associated with early intervention work, such as the detection of early warning signs, are also found in relapse prevention. Relapse prevention strategies were originally described in relation to alcohol addiction (Marlatt and Gordon, 1985) and have been expanded to cover a range of problems in which relapse can occur, for example substance abuse, gambling and offending. Relapse prevention encompasses a wide range of strategies that focus on reducing the risk of relapse. These are primarily cognitive and behavioural techniques, which focus on self-management. Relapse prevention is a self-control intervention which tries to enhance the person's own ability to change problematic thinking and behaviour, and to make lifestyle changes to reduce their chances of relapse.

The relapse prevention approach fits well with the vulnerability stress model as it helps clients to identify potential precipitating factors, focusing on enhancing skills to identify, anticipate and cope with high risk situations, identify sources of stress in their lifestyle, and develop and improve their overall coping capacity. Concepts such as high risk situations, that is, those situations or conditions that increase the risk of potential relapse, and identifying 'early warning signs' are particularly helpful. Whether or not the person has the ability to cope with high risk situations becomes a crucial factor in preventing relapse. The three main goals in relapse prevention work are increasing awareness, changing lifestyle and developing coping responses.

This approach has been used very successfully in the field of addictive behaviours, but, as yet, there has been little research on its effectiveness with schizophrenia. However, the current programme draws on key elements of this approach, in particular identifying, acting on and reducing factors which increase the chances of relapse.

In summary, a number of different psychological approaches and techniques have been developed to address the problems associated with schizophrenia. It is recognised that people with a diagnosis of schizophrenia are a very diverse group whose problems are often complex and multifactorial. No one intervention is therefore likely to address the variety of associated problems. There is a need for comprehensive treatment approaches drawing on 'what works' from a variety of sources. This programme attempts to bring together such approaches to provide clients with a broad-based selection of interventions and techniques within a supportive and collaborative therapeutic relationship.

The modular approach

It is recognised that interventions must be tailored to fit the individual's needs, their personal capabilities and their current strengths and abilities. This programme, while offering specific strategies, techniques and interventions, is flexible and designed to be used creatively and responsively. The number, length and frequency of sessions should be decided with the clients. The programme is divided into modules rather than individual sessions in order to maximise flexibility; however, suggested session plans are given with allocated time guidance in order to illustrate how modules might be presented. As a rough guide divisions into 1 hour 30-minute sessions are suggested. Session length should be determined by the needs of the clients and will also be influenced by the setting in which the intervention is offered. Hour-and-a-half sessions – even with tea breaks – will be too long for some clients and therefore two 45-minute sessions might be more appropriate. In practice the length of sessions will also be influenced by the number of clients in the group. Individual feedback and sharing of experiences will require more time the greater the number of group members.

Although essentially designed as a groupwork programme, there are a number of interventions which require clients to work on their own or in pairs with facilitator assistance. Some interventions should be carried out in additional one-to-one sessions.

The proposed number of sessions, excluding assessment sessions, is between 30 and 60 depending on the elected session length and number of individual supplementary sessions. Dependent on frequency of delivery the programme is approximately 6 to 12 months in duration. The National Institute for Clinical Excellence found that:

> longer treatments with cognitive behavioural therapy are significantly more effective than shorter ones, which may improve depressive symptoms but are unlikely to improve psychotic symptoms. An adequate course … should be of more than 6 months' duration and include more than ten planned sessions.
>
> *(NICE 2002)*

The suggested structure for each session is as follows:

1. Brief review of previous session
2. Overview of current session's content and aims
3. Main session intervention
4. Summary and question and answer time.

It is an artificial distinction to separate assessment from intervention. The first stage of the programme focuses on assessment, which can be a very useful tool in engaging the client and developing a mutual understanding. The assessment process can be as specific or as comprehensive as is required.

Module 1 focuses on engagement, treatment preparation, 'insight', self-efficacy, defining 'schizophrenia' and agreeing the language. It also has a strong educative component, providing information about diagnosis and a working model of schizophrenia.

Module 2 examines the individual's experiences and understanding of their diagnosis and how this has affected their life. Timelines are used to review the person's life. Personal identification of the onset, course and consequences of the 'illness' are examined. There is an emphasis on self-knowledge and coping.

Module 3 focuses on the positive symptoms of the diagnosis, presenting a cognitive behavioural model within which the individual's experiences can be explored. Specific symptoms such as delusional beliefs, paranoid thoughts, hallucinatory and other experiences are examined. The focus is on identification, understanding and coping with such experiences.

Module 4 aims to promote the person's protective factors in order to improve their ability to cope with the problems associated with their diagnosis. This includes identification of sources of stress and how to cope with stress, negative symptoms, interpersonal skills, problem solving and increasing self-efficacy. The role of medication and adherence to medication is also examined.

Module 5 brings together the main elements covered in the programme. Personalised relapse prevention plans are developed and future directions are explored.

Assessment

PART II

The research literature and published psychometrics related to the assessment of psychosis are extensive. That so much effort has been directed towards attempting to measure various aspects of psychosis is perhaps an indicator that it is an elusive and complex area. A handbook of assessment of psychosis published nearly a decade ago (Barnes and Nelson, 1994) details over 300 assessment instruments covering areas such as diagnosis, change in psychopathology, positive symptoms, thought disorder, negative symptoms, affective symptoms, cognitive functioning, suicidal risk, social functioning, aggression and insight.

The assessment of schizophrenia must be multifactorial; no one instrument is definitive in its assessment. As well as formal psychometric tools, there are a number of types of assessment, including behavioural observation, self-report, self-monitoring diaries and role play assessment. Information can also be collated from a number of sources: the clients themselves, carers, relatives, mental health professionals and case notes. A thorough assessment should contain formal and informal measures, quantitative and qualitative measures and information from a variety of sources.

The purpose of assessment

The selection of assessment method and choice of measures will be determined by the reasons for the assessment. In clinical settings the primary purposes of assessment are:

- To gain a full understanding of the person's experiences and an accurate record of their current problems. There are a number of areas which could be assessed to develop this understanding, including comprehensive symptomatology scales, interpersonal strengths and problems, coping and 'insight'.
- To monitor change over time. Change over time can be measured by ongoing monitoring procedures such as personal questionnaires, diaries, symptom rating questionnaires and behavioural records.
- To evaluate treatment effectiveness. Treatment effectiveness can be measured using assessments which are sensitive to change. Assessments that cover the range of associated symptoms are generally used to measure the effect of treatment. Any treatment, especially pharmacological treatments, may have deleterious as well as beneficial effects so measuring a range of symptoms helps to give a broader view of such effects, for example delusional beliefs might decrease, whereas

depression might increase. General symptomatology measures can also be useful in monitoring the course of the disorder over time. Choice of instrument will depend on the level of comprehensiveness required. Generally, the more comprehensive the measure the longer the administration time. The level of sensitivity to change is also an important factor. The most sensitive will include measures of intensity, frequency or distress rather than, for example, absent/present ratings. Effectiveness can also be measured by clients' self-ratings of treatment satisfaction and perceived usefulness of treatment.

- Assessment as an intervention. Assessment itself can be a helpful form of intervention. The analysis of a person's understanding and recognition of problems, that is, 'insight' can serve as a measure of change, but is also useful in engagement and developing a therapeutic relationship. Likewise, self-monitoring by use of symptom diaries can help a person to identify variations in their symptoms and thus reinforce the idea that such symptoms are not fixed and stable features. Assessment of coping abilities can serve to highlight areas of success and to enhance self-efficacy. Similarly many of the interventions described in subsequent modules, such as time line analysis and individual analysis of symptoms, can also be helpful assessments.

Assessment measures

The following synopsis outlines a variety of potentially useful tools for assessment. It is not intended as a recommended assessment package, but rather describes several measures which might be selected to suit the required purpose. It is suggested that no more than three or four measures are used prior to starting any intervention, and that these include 'before and after' evaluation measures. Other measures can be used during the course of the programme, when appropriate, for example, drug attitudes scales when addressing medication issues, and interpersonal problems inventory when covering protective factors.

Comprehensive assessment of symptomatology

Present State Examination (PSE) (Wing et al, 1974)

This commonly used interview schedule takes approximately 2 hours to complete, and was developed as a diagnostic tool for psychiatric illnesses. It consists of 54 standard questions and several supplementary questions. Identified symptoms are rated as either moderate or severe. A variety of symptoms are covered including depression, anxiety, concentration problems, delusions and hallucinations. It assesses symptoms experienced within the previous month. The authors recommend that the PSE should be administered by trained raters.

Brief Psychiatric Rating Scale (BPRS) (Overall and Gorham, 1962)

This is a very widely used scale, perhaps due to its brevity. It takes between 15 and 30 minutes to administer. There are 16 'symptom constructs' which are rated on a seven-point severity scale. The symptoms, however, are difficult to differentiate and often do not describe the client's problems.

Comprehensive Psychopathological Rating Scale (CPRS)
(Asberg et al, 1978)

This scale comprises 67 items and takes approximately an hour to complete. The items include both reported symptoms and behavioural observation, and were selected as being sensitive to change. Ratings are made of severity and frequency.

Assessment of positive and negative symptoms

While comprehensive rating scales for psychosis include both positive symptoms and negative symptoms, the measures are often unspecific and merely rate for the presence or absence of such symptoms, or elicit a general severity rating. Scales which cover a variety of positive and negative symptoms in more detail include the *Positive And Negative Syndrome Scale* (PANSS) (Kay et al, 1989), the *Scale for the Assessment of Positive Symptoms* (SAPS) (Andreasen, 1984) and the *Scale for the Assessment of Negative Symptoms* (SANS) (Andreasen, 1981). These scales can be used to assess the presence and severity of a range of specific symptoms, and yield more detailed information than comprehensive rating scales.

The PANSS and SANS can provide a formal measure of a range of negative symptoms. As negative symptoms represent an absence of emotion or behaviour, such as emotional unresponsiveness, flattened affect and poverty of speech, they can be difficult to measure. Also, with negative symptoms in particular, the observer's judgement often does not concur with the client's own reported difficulties. Thus while clinician ratings can be useful to gauge overt negative symptoms and to monitor change in such symptoms, a client's self-report is more likely to identify areas which the client would like to address.

Subjective Experience of Deficits in Schizophrenia (SEDS) (Liddle and Barnes, 1988) measures the client's own experience of negative symptoms. The SEDS is a semi-structured interview, which rates 21 items on a five-point scale. The categories include abnormal thinking, disturbance of affect, motivation, disturbance of perception and intolerance of stress. This scale is helpful in that it rates not only the occurrence of the experience but also the perceived disruption, the degree of distress and overall severity.

The current programme focuses on the importance of mutually agreed treatment goals and enhancing the person's ability to manage their symptoms and reduce the associated distress of target symptoms. The most personally relevant and useful assessment procedure for clients are those that use tailored self-rating scales constructed by the therapist with the client.

Personal questionnaires (PQ)

Personal questionnaire techniques were originally described by Shapiro (1961). The technique has been creatively modified for positive symptoms of schizophrenia, in particular delusions, and this is now an established and proficient assessment and monitoring procedure (Garety, 1985; Brett-Jones et al, 1987). These scales comprise individually constructed written statements, which rate for example the conviction and preoccupation of personal delusional beliefs. The technique is flexible, and any pertinent aspects of the symptoms can be added and monitored, for example distress ratings or perceived coping. Ratings can be made by the client using numerical or visual analogue scales. Personal questionnaires are sensitive to small changes over repeated measures, and therefore provide a structured but individually tailored self-report scale. Examples of personal questionnaires are presented in Module 3.

Beliefs About Voices Questionnaire (BAVQ) (Chadwick and Birchwood, 1995)

This is a more formal 30-item questionnaire which measures various aspects of a person's beliefs about their auditory hallucinations. It measures malevolence (six items), benevolence (six items), resistance (nine items), engagement (eight items) and power (one item). This questionnaire is useful in drawing out the personal significance of the person's voices, and facilitates examination of the connection between the content of beliefs and the individual's personal history. The questionnaire provides a detailed basis from which to develop an understanding of clients' views. Such information, as well as indicating possible treatment avenues, can also be used to gauge change.

Assessment of depression

Depression can go undetected in people with a diagnosis of schizophrenia because symptoms such as social withdrawal, poverty of speech and anhedonia are often interpreted as negative symptoms whereas they are also common symptoms of depression.

Medication side effects can also mimic depressive symptoms, for example lack of facial expression, loss of spontaneity and paucity of gesture.

Institutionalisation can also lead to lack of spontaneity, reduced motivation and volition. Thus negative symptoms, medication side effects, the effects of institutionalisation and depression can be difficult to differentiate, and careful assessment is needed to help clarify the nature of such difficulties.

Depression is common in people with a diagnosis of schizophrenia. As many as 50 per cent of people discharged from hospital with a diagnosis of schizophrenia reported depressive symptoms at follow up (Falloon et al, 1978). Depressive symptoms are common in the early stages or prodromal phase in first episodes of acute schizophrenia and are also early predictors of impending relapse (Herz and Melville, 1980). Recognition of symptoms such as reduced appetite, sleep disturbance and depressed mood can therefore be valuable early warning signs to a potential relapse. Depression can also be caused by the experiences associated with having a diagnosis of schizophrenia, including hospitalisation and loss of friends and/or employment. It has been suggested that neuroleptic medication side effects, as well as mimicking some depressive symptoms, might actually cause depression (Ananth and Ghadirian, 1980).

There are no scales developed specifically to assess depressive symptoms in people with a diagnosis of schizophrenia; however, several depression rating scales are widely available such as the *Beck Depression Inventory* (BDI) (Beck et al, 1961). This self-rating scale is quick and easy to complete and is very widely used. The *Hamilton Rating Scale for Depression* (HRSD) (Hamilton, 1960) is another commonly used observer rating scale which measures severity of depression.

Assessment of interpersonal problems

People with a diagnosis of schizophrenia often have specific difficulties in relating to other people for a variety of reasons. These include distraction and interference by acute symptoms, reactions of others to perceived social difficulties, loss of confidence and sensitivity to stress. An assessment of interpersonal problems is therefore helpful in eliciting current difficulties in this area, both as an indicator of treatment focus and as a measure of change.

The Inventory of Interpersonal Problems (IIP-32) (Barkham et al, 1996)

This is a short version of the *Inventory of Interpersonal Problems, Psychometric Properties and Clinical Applications* (IIPPPCA) (Horowitz et al, 1988). It is intended for use with people with a range of mental health problems, and is suitable for those with a diagnosis of schizophrenia. It comprises eight subscales, with each question being scored on a five-point scale, and covers the areas of assertiveness, sociability, supportiveness, caring, dependency, regression, involvement and openness. It is brief, easy to use, assesses a range of interpersonal problems and is sensitive to change.

Assessment of social anxiety

In common with many people, those with a diagnosis of schizophrenia can find social situations particularly difficult or anxiety arousing. People often feel tense in unfamiliar situations and avoid talking to people, worry what people might be thinking of them, and so on. These concerns are often particularly pronounced in people with mental health problems, and can be exacerbated by feelings of suspiciousness, paranoid beliefs and experiences of social exclusion.

Two scales designed to measure social difficulties in the general population are the 30-item *Fear of Negative Evaluation* scale (FNE) and the 28-item *Social Avoidance and Distress* scale (SAD) (Watson and Friend, 1969). Both are self-report questionnaires which require a true or false answer to a list of statements.

People scoring highly on the FNE scale tend to become nervous in evaluative situations and try to avoid disapproval or gain the approval of others. Those high on the SAD scale tend to avoid social interactions, prefer to work alone, talk less, worry about and are less confident in social situations. These scales are helpful in indicating possible problem areas to be addressed as they highlight particular social anxieties and fears, which can be explored and incorporated into treatment plans (see Module 4). These scales can also provide a measure of treatment change.

Assessment of self-esteem

Being diagnosed as having a severe mental illness, and the subsequent social, personal and occupational implications of this often lead to low self-esteem, loss of confidence and loss of feelings of self-worth and competence.

Self-esteem comprises several components and incorporates a sense of personal worthiness, physical appearance, social competence and power. The self-concept questionnaire (Robson, 1989) is a 30-item self-report scale that includes questions on significance, worthiness, appearance, social acceptability, resilience and determination, competence, control over personal destiny and value of existence. Ratings are on an eight-point Likert scale. This measure can give an indication of the degree of self-esteem problems as well as providing a measure of change.

Insight

Traditional views of insight into psychosis give great emphasis to the importance of increasing the insight of the person into their mental illness. In essence there are three components of insight commonly described: acceptance of the need for treatment (primarily medication); recognition of having a mental illness; and recognition that their positive symptoms are indeed symptoms of illness and not real phenomena (David, 1990). However, this is a very restrictive view of insight, therefore traditional schedules or measures of insight are not used. An alternative psychological interpretation of insight is more fully described in Module 1.

Psychological Intervention Programme

PART III

MODULE 1

Engagement and treatment preparation

Overview of Module

- Setting the scene
- Establishing group rules
- Introduction to the programme
- Agreeing the language
- How schizophrenia is diagnosed
- A psychological model of schizophrenia
- Psychological insight
- Treatment preparation
- Self-efficacy
- Personal aims

Suggested Session Plans

Introductions/icebreakers	**10 min**
Hopes and fears	**10 min**
Group rules	**10 min**
Introduction to the programme	**1 hour**
Agreeing the language	**15 min**
How schizophrenia is diagnosed	**20 min**
Personal views of diagnosis	**40 min**
Information giving	**15 min**
Psychological model	**1 hour**
Reflection and personal relevance of model	**30 min**

What is insight?	**20 min**
Personal experiences and discussion	**30 min**
Agreeing a working definition	**10 min**
Case example and discussion	**30 min**
Treatment preparation exploratory discussion	**15 min**
Case example	**10 min**
Treatment experiences discussion	**20 min**
Self-efficacy exploration	**20 min**
Case example	**10 min**
Personal aims	**15 min**

Setting the scene

Intervention begins the first time you meet the client. The first stages involve engagement, that is, getting to know the person, what they want, if anything, from treatment, their expectations, their previous experience and so on. This is done by talking and listening to the person!

Clients, particularly those with no previous experience of group work, are likely to have some concerns about undertaking such a programme. They are likely to feel anxious, nervous and possibly suspicious. The initial sessions should, therefore, be as relaxed and informal as possible while maintaining a sense of the importance of the work.

It is worth spending time creating a positive physical environment in which the groupwork can take place. Although this can be difficult in some mental health institutions it is worth paying attention to the lighting, temperature and arrangement of furniture. A circle of comfortable chairs unrestricted by tables is best. Further ambience can be added by the use of aromatherapy oils.

There are several facilitative exercises or 'ice-breakers' which can be used to help clients to feel more comfortable within a group. Introductions can be made more 'interactive' by dividing the group into pairs. Clients are given two to three minutes to tell their partner their name and two things about themselves, such as a hobby or interest; clients then introduce their partner to the group using the information imparted to them.

Group members should be encouraged to express their feelings, hopes and fears about the group. In pairs clients should be invited to tell their partner about their fears and anxieties about the group. Repeat the exercise, this time sharing some of their hopes and expectations of the group. Clients should then be encouraged to feedback their hopes and fears to the group. These can be listed on a flipchart.

Establishing group rules

Group rules are vital in order to help establish a feeling of safety and containment within the group and to promote group cohesion.

The rules should be made by the group members themselves, with all suggestions being discussed by the group and included only if all agree. These can be written on a flipchart and later produced as a handout for all members to sign and keep as their personal copy; a colour printer and laminator make them look particularly good.

An example of a group rules contract is presented in Handout 1 'Group Rules Contract', and a sample 'group rules' list is shown in Box 1.

BOX 1 Group rules

I will arrive on time and will remain for the duration of the group
I will respect the confidentiality of the group (what is said in the group stays in the group)
I will expect to be shown respect and will respect others in the group
I will try to be open and honest
I will not interrupt when others are talking and will listen to what people say
I will try to be helpful to others

In the first session provide each person with a folder in which to file their handouts and worksheets.

Introduction to the programme

How the person views therapy is critical. Examination of the important ingredients of successful therapies suggests that one of the most important preconditions is that the client has positive expectations (Prochaska and Di Clemente, 1982). Other preconditions, according to the authors, are motivation to change and a warm and trusting therapeutic relationship.

The first sessions should, therefore, focus on explaining the proposed treatment programme, eliciting people's views about it, and promoting positive expectations. Handout 2 'All about the programme' provides a brief summary of the programme. This should form the basis of a discussion and question and answer session.

Having explained the nature and content of the programme and answered queries and concerns ask group members for their views and opinions about the programme. Questions should include:

- How relevant does this type of programme seem to you?
- Do you think that the programme is likely to be beneficial for you?
- How confident are you that taking part in this programme is a good idea?

Ensure that each member of the group is encouraged to give their opinion and feels that their views are heard.

Agreeing the language

The people participating in this programme will all have been given a diagnosis of schizophrenia at some point. Some may disagree with their diagnosis, believe that they have a different type of mental health problem or disagree that they are suffering from any form of mental illness. Often, despite being in the mental health system for some years, people have not had the opportunity for a full and open discussion about their diagnosis and its implications. People with a diagnosis of schizophrenia usually have some preconceptions and understanding about the diagnosis. They might have little factual knowledge or may even have received misinformation from prior contacts with psychiatric services. The traditional lay view of schizophrenia, as a mental illness or madness which takes over the person completely and renders them insane, or producing a 'split personality,' is still widely held. The medical view of schizophrenia as an illness with strong genetic and neurobiological components, which produces bizarre delusions and hallucinations that require medication is also common. People with the diagnosis, therefore, are often fearful of what it means, realise the stigma associated with it, and hold misconceptions about its nature, course and treatment. The term 'schizophrenia' can therefore evoke strong feelings, and a discussion should be held to agree the terminology to be used during the programme. Alternatives might include 'mental illness', mental disorder', 'mental health problems' or simply 'difficulties'.

How schizophrenia is diagnosed

While clients might disagree with their diagnosis, most are interested to know how such a diagnosis was made, and therefore a brief summary of DSM-IV or ICD-10 diagnostic criteria should be presented.

An outline of how diagnoses are made should be presented as follows: the *Diagnostic and Statistical Manual*, DSM-IV-TR (American Psychiatric Association, 2000) details the criteria which should be met in order to make a diagnosis of all recognised psychiatric disorders. For schizophrenia five main criteria must be fulfilled:

- First, at least one of a list of positive symptoms must be present.
- Second, a decline in level of functioning must be apparent.
- Third, there must be a duration of continuous signs of illness for at least 6 months at some point in the person's life.

- The fourth criterion excludes related mental disorders such as schizoaffective disorder.
- The fifth excludes any organic disorder.

These criteria were produced by a panel of experts and compiled with the principal goal of usefulness, reliability and acceptability to clinicians and researchers. The DSM has been revised and updated from its original form over several decades, and its current criteria are likely to be further modified in the future.

The *International Classification of Diseases 10* (ICD-10) (WHO, 1993) is a classification of mental and behavioural disorders. There are over 300 disorders described, with detailed clinical descriptions and diagnostic guidelines. The original manual was conceived in the 1960s, when the Mental Health Programme of the World Health Organization (WHO) attempted to improve the diagnosis and classification of mental disorders. Following a comprehensive consultation process of psychiatrists in a variety of countries, the results were published in guidelines (ICD-8). These were developed and expanded using professional seminars, workshops and reviews; 'field trials' were also carried out. The current tenth edition contains a set of criteria and assessment instruments which help in the classification of disorders. For each disorder a description is given of the main clinical features, and any associated features. Diagnostic guidelines are provided of the number and nature of symptoms required to make a diagnosis. However, there is still a large degree of 'clinical judgement' and the concept of 'confident provisional and tentative' diagnoses is raised. The ICD-10 states:

> these descriptions and guidelines carry no theoretical implications as they do not pretend to be comprehensive statements about the current state of knowledge of the disorders. They are simply a set of symptoms and comments that have been agreed by a large number of advisors and consultants in many different countries, to be a reasonable basis for defining the limits of categories in the classification of mental disorders.
>
> *World Health Organization, 1992*

Handout 3 'How schizophrenia is diagnosed' should be distributed to aid discussion.

This discussion should include asking the clients how they think their diagnosis of schizophrenia was made, that is, which particular symptoms or criteria might have been used. Encourage clients to complete Worksheet 1 'How my diagnosis was made', providing individual assistance as required. Note that clients are not necessarily expected to agree with their diagnosis but merely to think about how the doctor made the diagnosis, that is, what evidence they used in order to decide on a diagnosis of schizophrenia.

Ask clients whether they agree with their diagnosis and, if not, why they do not agree. Finally, lead a discussion to elicit how clients feel about having such a diagnosis. There is likely to be a wide variety of responses to this varying from denial of mental health problems to feeling relieved at the acknowledgement that their frightening experiences are common symptoms of a recognised mental disorder.

There is much literature available on schizophrenia, and this should be provided to suit the needs and requests of each individual. This might range from recommending books on schizophrenia, leaflets produced by the National Schizophrenia Fellowship or providing basic facts. Handout 4 'Fact file' provides basic information, which can be elaborated by discussion.

A psychological model of schizophrenia

Presenting a psychological model of schizophrenia provides a framework which can help to demystify and normalise the concept. The model demonstrates that 'schizophrenia' is not merely a medical condition but that it is influenced by social, psychological and environmental factors. The key point in the presentation of this model is that as there are many factors involved in exacerbating symptoms and problems, there are also many ways to help alleviate the difficulties. The model presented in Handout 5 'A psychological model of schizophrenia' is a simplified version of the vulnerability stress model (Neuchterlein and Dawson, 1984), which was described in detail in Part I.

The model can be presented on a flipchart or overhead prjector slide, with an explanation of the model as follows.

There are several components to this model, the most important is that there is an interaction between a person's proneness or 'vulnerability' to develop schizophrenia, and the life circumstances or environmental influences that the person experiences.

Personal proneness is likely to involve at least three factors. The first is the way a person makes sense of information received from their senses. This is called information processing. The five senses – seeing, hearing, tasting, feeling and smelling – provide us with information about our environment. This information is passed to the brain; the brain interprets the information, matching the new information with previous experiences. We interpret, classify and organise such information, and then make decisions about how to respond. We are all prone to make mistakes in information processing, and people with a proneness to schizophrenia might have specific predispositions to such errors.

Second, our personality; the type of person we are might also influence the development of schizophrenia. People who tend to withdraw from social contact, or be difficult to get to know, might have a predisposition towards developing schizophrenia. There are a number of personality characteristics that are commonly found in children who go on to receive a diagnosis of schizophrenia later in life. They tend to be more introverted and withdrawn, and prefer to spend time on their own rather than with others.

Third, the autonomic nervous system, which controls the body's responses to stress, might be more reactive in people who develop schizophrenia.

Although some people have a predisposition to develop schizophrenia because of physiological, genetic and biological factors, this does not mean such problems are insurmountable. There are several protective factors which can reduce the impact of vulnerability factors, including the person's ability to cope. The more able a person is to manage problems and difficulties, the more likely they are to reduce the influence of underlying vulnerabilities. Self-efficacy is one's ability to tackle problems and take control of situations. Improving coping abilities and self-efficacy are central to becoming more resilient.

Another major protective factor is antipsychotic medication. There have been many advances in producing effective medication that can alleviate the symptoms of schizophrenia.

Stressful life events, such as divorce, losing a job or the death of someone close, are factors which affect our mental health. While stressful life events happen to everyone at some point in their lives, some people are less able to cope than others. Sudden increases in stress might contribute to an emergence of symptoms of schizophrenia.

Difficult and stressful living conditions also influence our mental health. Ongoing stress, such as noise, day-to-day hassles and demands which are hard to meet, can induce high levels of stress.

A third source of environmental stress is from other people. Critical or emotionally overinvolved attitudes of others, particularly those close to us, have been found to be a particularly significant sources of stress.

Some people are better able to withstand the stressors in their lives. Those who have good social support and are good at solving problems seem to do best. There are a number of psychological and social solutions to help deal with life events, daily stress and the impact of other people. These can be helpful in protecting against the influence of environmental stressors.

The interaction of 'vulnerabilities' and 'protectors' will lead to a number of possible outcomes. As vulnerability factors increase, the greater the likelihood is of experiencing a period of mental health problems or an acute episode of schizophrenia. However, the greater the protective factors, the less likely the person is to experience such symptoms. Outcomes of course also include the person's ability to function in a variety of ways, including social, occupational and personal functioning. The more effective a person's coping abilities, self-efficacy and support, the more likely they are to be able to function in these areas, and to minimise the effect of their predisposition.

Following this explanation allow plenty of time for group members to ask questions, comment on the model and reflect on the personal relevance of this information.

Psychological insight

The commonest recorded sign or symptom associated with a diagnosis of schizophrenia is 'lack of insight' (WHO, 1973). People with a diagnosis of schizophrenia are frequently in conflict with mental health professionals regarding the issue of 'insight'. Unfortunately, it remains widely accepted that people with a diagnosis of schizophrenia often do not have the ability to perceive their difficulties accurately. The concept of insight is often poorly understood and viewed as a dichotomous characteristic, that is, either being present or absent. Insight is also viewed as a stable characteristic. However, this absolutist, rigid view has been challenged by studies which examine people's understanding of their disorder and the ability of many people to give accurate and reliable retrospective accounts of the onset and course of their symptoms.

One of the most significant consequences for people with a diagnosis of schizophrenia, that of mental health professionals judging their level of insight as poor, is that this often heralds a breakdown in communication, with clients feeling misunderstood and professionals thinking the person is incapable of understanding. Psychiatrists tend to hold the view described by David (1990), that is, insight is composed of three distinct but overlapping dimensions: the recognition that one has a mental illness; treatment compliance; and the ability to relabel unusual mental events, such as delusions, as pathological. That is, people are described as insightful if they accept the traditional medical model of psychosis. However, if insight is removed from its restrictive medical definition to a psychological interpretation of the concept, it can become the basis for engagement and development of a mutually agreed formulation of the person's difficulties; that is, psychological insight as self-understanding and recognition of abilities and problems. Broadening the three proposed components of insight to take into consideration the person's own perspective as psychologically valid and meaningful to them, provides a basis for arriving at mutually agreed treatment goals.

A helpful way of starting a discussion about insight is to ask the clients to brainstorm the question: 'What is insight?' Typical responses include those presented in Box 2.

BOX 2 What is insight?

Knowing about yourself
Understanding your illness
Thinking normally
Agreeing with the doctors
Knowing that you are ill
Taking medication
Realising your problems

This can then lead to a discussion about personal experiences of insight/ lack of insight asking people to recall if mental health professionals and family members or friends have ever disagreed with them about whether or not they have a mental illness, their possible need for medication and the view that their unusual experiences might be signs of pathological illness.

This brief exercise is often very illuminating in terms of past or current experiences of feeling alienated and disbelieved, and can illustrate how other people's reactions can further exacerbate the difficulties caused by 'psychotic symptoms'.

The desired outcome of this session is to arrive at a mutually agreed working definition of psychological insight, for example insight as a shared understanding of what the problems are and how to deal with them.

The following case example illustrates that 'lack of insight' is not a barrier to treatment, and also that often 'insight' as a goal of treatment is not helpful to the client. Rather, reaching a mutually agreed treatment goal is likely to be very beneficial.

In the initial sessions it is particularly valuable to present case examples to illustrate how a psychological approach to treatment has been helpful to clients. Use sample case examples or examples from your own interventions suitably anonymised to maintain confidentiality.

Case example

DAVID was a 24-year-old man with a diagnosis of schizophrenia/persistent delusional disorder. He believed that the police had conspired to 'set him up' and incriminate him in a number of crimes, which he had not committed, over several years. This was a very strongly held belief, which persisted in spite of any evidence of police actions against him. The belief persisted over four years, despite many trials of antipsychotic medication and individual treatment aimed at challenging them. David was often described in his medical notes as having 'total lack of insight'. Thus the treatment goal of improving insight failed to produce any effect over a considerable period of attempted intervention.

David was then seen by a psychologist. Discussion with David about the underlying feelings that the belief engendered was more fruitful. He described feeling victimised and ridiculed. This left him feeling depressed, hopeless and angry. Previous interventions, where he viewed the professionals as disbelieving him and implying that he was wrong, had further entrenched his belief that people were against him. Indeed he had started to believe that the professionals involved were also part of the police conspiracy against him. The agreed treatment goal, therefore, was to reduce the negative subjective experience of holding such beliefs. David and his therapist agreed that the belief may or may not be accurate, but that the effect of holding such a belief was having a detrimental effect on him and reducing his ability to cope. Intervention therefore focused not on challenging the belief but on changing the associated thoughts and feelings. The outcome of such a focus is summarised below.

Previous belief:	Police have set me up, they want to destroy me.
Resultant thoughts:	They are winning. They are humiliating me. I am a victim.
Associated feelings:	Depressed, hopeless, angry.
Resultant behaviour:	Planning revenge, efforts to expose conspiracy.

Intervention – six sessions discussing associated thoughts and feelings, and coping strategies.

Current belief:	Police have set me up. They want to destroy me.
Resultant thoughts:	I won't let them beat me. I won't let them ruin my life any more. 'What's done is done.'
Associated feelings:	Relieved, in control.
Behaviour:	Not preoccupied with revenge, focusing on other plans.

Thus although the belief remained unchanged, the effect of the belief was considerably changed, resulting in an improved ability to cope, a considerable reduction in distress and a significant reduction in the level of preoccupation with the belief.

Treatment preparation

Examining the person's beliefs and attitudes about potential treatments is very important. It is likely that their beliefs will be based on previous experience of treatment interventions, as well as on their view of whether their problems are indeed 'treatable'. Attitudes vary from absolute pessimism of 'nothing works' to unrealistic optimism of treatment as a 'cure'. Proposed exploratory questions to assist in discussing attitude towards treatment are presented in Box 3.

Understanding a person's views and beliefs about treatment also provides an opportunity to discuss their concerns and to address any misconceptions. Often people who have previously been seen as resistant to interventions can be motivated to accept treatment by addressing their underlying beliefs, and finding a 'way in' which fits with their view of their difficulties.

BOX 3 Proposed schedule for exploring 'insight', treatment preparation and self-efficacy

Acceptance of mental health problem	◦ In your opinion do you have a mental health health problem? ◦ Do you think mental health services can help you in any way? ◦ How do you explain your (unusual beliefs/ voices/visions/other phenomena)? ◦ Have you previously had mental health problems? ◦ Do you know anyone with mental health problems? How do you know when they are not well?
Treatment preparation	◦ Do you think it might be worthwhile to work on improving your problems associated with your diagnosis? ◦ Do you have any concerns about psychological treatment? ◦ How reasonable does this type of therapy seem to you? ◦ What are your previous experiences of treatment? ◦ What would you like to get out of treatment?
Self-efficacy	◦ Do you have some ideas about how to manage your mental health problems? ◦ What have you found helpful in the past? ◦ Do you notice any changes in your symptoms over time? ◦ Does anything make the symptoms worse/better? ◦ Can you recognise when you are becoming mentally unwell?

The following case example could be used to illustrate the importance of finding a treatment approach that is meaningful.

Case example

A YOUNG MAN with an interest in science and technology holds the opinion that 'psychological treatment is pointless because I have a medical condition due to a chemical imbalance, and talking about it does not help'. Offering the opportunity to 'test out' this hypothesis as a 'behavioural experiment' was acceptable to him and provided him with an opportunity to use psychological interventions. He was motivated in this way to carry on with what he had previously seen as 'just talking'. He began to appreciate the notion that his mental state did indeed change over time by completing simple mood rating scales. He came to understand that his mental state was often influenced by external factors, such as stress, and was therefore amenable to change. He viewed this as stress exacerbating the chemical imbalance, and became engaged in trying to reduce this, with some success.

Lead a group discussion on what makes treatment 'meaningful' to each client. Encourage the use of examples – positive and negative – from previous experiences.

Self-efficacy

Bandura's (1977) influential social learning theory known as the Self-efficacy Theory, examines the role of people's expectations in treatment and the effect of such cognitions on behaviour. The basic proposition is that behavioural change by treatment is mediated by a cognitive mechanism: 'efficacy expectations', that is, the judgement that one has the ability to carry out a certain behaviour. Bandura proposed that any intervention is effective only to the extent that it increases the person's expectations of personal efficacy.

Having a diagnosis of schizophrenia can result in feeling helpless, powerless and overwhelmed. Self-efficacy can restore feelings of control, help the person to feel less distressed by their symptoms and instil hope that they can improve their mental health despite having such a diagnosis. Having an expectation of self-determination does not imply that the person is responsible for the course and outcome of their disorder, but that they can help to reduce the consequences of such a disorder. Self-efficacy in relation to the management of psychotic symptoms has been described as having three phases (Breier and Strauss, 1983). First, the person becomes aware of the existence of psychotic or pre-psychotic behaviour by self-monitoring. Secondly, they recognise the implications of these behaviours as a signal of the disorder, and third, mechanisms of self-control are used, for example, self-instruction. Emphasis on previous and current coping skills and competence can improve feelings of self-efficacy and help to motivate people to participate in self-management.

Present the following case example to illustrate the importance of using personal knowledge.

Case example

SARAH, a woman with a history of repeated hospital admissions, was referred for psychological assessment. Her medical notes described her relapses as 'rapid and dramatic', however, by detailed assessment she was in fact able to describe many early warning signs (prodrome). However, she disclosed that she feared hospitalisation and therefore did not report any symptoms to her doctor. Treatment focused on her good ability to recognise early warning signs, and increasing her sense of self-efficacy. This led to the proposition that self-monitoring and early reporting to her doctor might enable interventions such as an increase in medication, which could reduce the necessity for hospitalisation.

Box 3 earlier lists some example questions to encourage discussion of self-efficacy.

Personal aims

In order to facilitate engagement and to assist in tailoring the programme to suit individual needs, each client should be encouraged to identify their personal aims.

This should be done individually, with assistance from facilitators as necessary. Provide clients with Worksheet 2 'My personal aims', on which to record their aims. Once completed each group member should feedback their aims to the group.

MODULE 1

Group rules contract

'Name of group'

Location ______________________

Day ______________________

Time ______________________

Group members ______________________

____

____

____

____

____

____

Group facilitators ______________________

____

Our rules
- ______________________
- ______________________
- ______________________
- ______________________
- ______________________
- ______________________
- ______________________

Signed ______________________ Date ______________________

All about the programme

(page 1 of 2)

This programme has three main aims:

1 To increase your knowledge and understanding of yourself and your mental health problems so that you can gain greater control of your life and what happens to you.
2 To help you cope more effectively with any problems you may experience, including those directly related to mental health and those which are a consequence of having a diagnosis of schizophrenia.
3 To improve your lifestyle and life skills in any areas which you think would be beneficial, such as coping with stress, improving communication and so on.

You are the expert on your own life; by reviewing your life, your coping abilities and what you have found to be helpful or unhelpful in the past, together we will be able to find ways of solving current problems and improve your ability to cope with problems in the future.

There are five modules which cover the following areas.

Module 1: Engagement and treatment preparation

- Helps you to get to know each other
- Explains the programme and what it covers
- Explores how a diagnosis of schizophrenia is made
- Introduces a psychological model of schizophrenia
- Orientates you to the programme and how you can be involved in your own treatment

Module 2: Individual analysis of person and 'schizophrenia'

- Focuses on you and your life so far, and looks at how schizophrenia has impacted on your life

All about the programme

(page 2 of 2)

- Examines the phases of schizophrenia and helps you identify and understand the course of your mental health problems
- Explores how your own experiences fit in with the phases of schizophrenia
- Helps you to identify and respond to early warning signs of mental health problems
- Explores how to reduce the impact of schizophrenia on your life

Module 3: Understanding and managing positive symptoms

- Examines the various interventions for 'positive' symptoms of schizophrenia
- Examines how to identify 'positive' symptoms and how to monitor them
- Explores ways of reducing distress caused by symptoms and how to use coping strategies effectively
- Provides psychological explanations of 'positive' symptoms
- Presents ways of modifying symptoms

Module 4: Maximising mental health

- Focuses on ways of increasing your 'protection' against future mental health problems
- Examines how to improve your interactions with other people
- Presents ways of coping with stress
- Examines negative symptoms and how to manage them
- Explores how to get the most out of medication

Module 5: Bringing it all together

- Reviews the key areas covered
- Explores future directions

How schizophrenia is diagnosed (page 1 of 2)

Schizophrenia is a very diverse and varied mental disorder. It is usually diagnosed by the presence of one or more of the following types of experiences:

- The belief that thoughts are being put into your head or taken out, or that other people can hear your thoughts.
- The belief that you are being influenced or controlled by something that has power over you, or you see or hear things that have special meanings for you.
- Hearing voices that others do not hear. They might comment on your behaviour or talk about you among themselves. The voices might be insulting, or might tell you what to do.
- Holding unusual beliefs about yourself which other people do not think are possible, for example thinking that you have superhuman powers or are a religious or political leader.

A diagnosis of schizophrenia might be made if you experience two or more of the following:

- Unusual or strange beliefs together with persistent hallucinations of any kind; hallucinations can include hearing, seeing, feeling, tasting or smelling things that other people do not.
- Breaks or intrusions in your train of thought which make it difficult to speak clearly or coherently, this might include making up new words or phrases.

How schizophrenia is diagnosed (page 2 of 2)

- Behaving in an unusual way, for example being very excitable or very lethargic or not talking.
- 'Negative' symptoms such as apathy, having little expression or feeling about things.
- A significant change in your behaviour, for example losing interest in work, social activities, not mixing with others, being self-absorbed or neglecting yourself.

These experiences must have been present for at least one month.

How my diagnosis was made

For use in conjunction with Handout 3 'How schizophrenia is diagnosed'

You might not agree with your diagnosis. However, in this exercise just think about how the doctor made the diagnosis. What evidence did he or she use?

Which symptoms or signs do you think were used to reach the diagnosis?

Consider the following:

- Any unusual or 'strange' beliefs
- Any experiences which other people do not experience, such as seeing things, hearing things that others do not
- Difficulties thinking
- Any unusual behaviour

Fact file (page 1 of 2)

How common?

- About one person in 100 is likely to receive a diagnosis of schizophrenia.
- 100,000 to 500,000 people in the UK today are likely to have been given a diagnosis of schizophrenia.

Does gender make a difference?

- Most men who develop the problems that lead to a diagnosis of schizophrenia do so before the age of 25. Women tend to develop such problems by age 30, but there is a wide variation.

Why me?

- Some people are more vulnerable to developing a psychotic disorder than others, you are more likely:
  — If you have a relative with the same or similar diagnosis
  — If you have experienced significant stress or trauma
  — If you have particular psychological, social or biological factors which are likely to contribute to a 'predisposition'

Fact file (page 2 of 2)

Treatment

- The most common form of help is medication. This is not a 'cure' but can help to alleviate or prevent symptoms
- Psychological treatments based on understanding the range of problems associated with a diagnosis of schizophrenia and enhancing coping abilities. There are many psychological interventions that can help to reduce the impact of serious mental health problems, lessen symptoms and reduce the chances and severity of relapse. Psychological treatments also help to improve awareness and understanding of problems and to develop successful coping strategies

Course

- As many as one-third of people with a diagnosis of schizophrenia recover completely after one 'psychotic' episode
- Some people experience 'relapses' in symptoms but remain symptom-free between these episodes
- Less than 25 per cent of people remain continuously affected.

A psychological model of schizophrenia

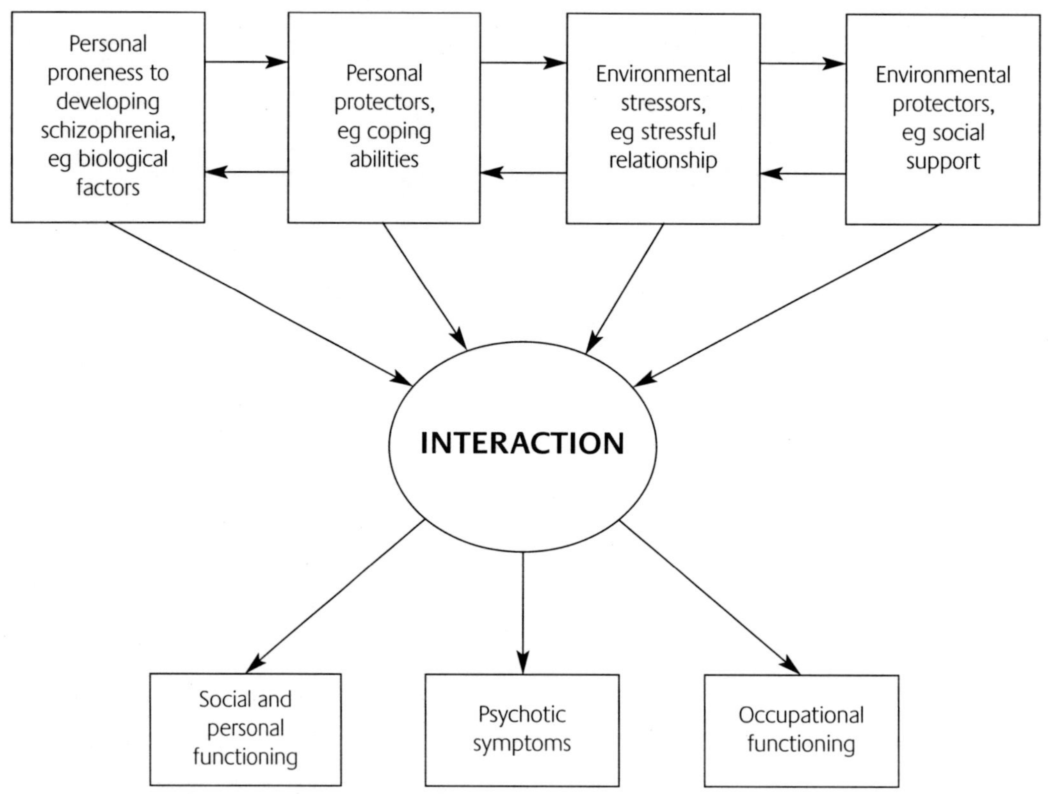

My personal aims

Use this sheet to record your personal aims, that is, what you would like to get out of participating in this programme. Consider what you would like to learn more about, things you would like to work on and things you would like to achieve.

MODULE 2

Individual analysis of person and 'schizophrenia'

Overview of Module

- Introduction
- About me
- Timeline: my life so far
- The phases of schizophrenia
- My prodrome: identification and responses
- My acute phase
- My remission/recovery phase
- My potential relapse phase
- Responding to relapse signs
- Living with schizophrenia: reducing the impact

Suggested Sessions Plan

Introduction	**10 min**
What I am like exercise	**35 min**
Discussion of personal changes	**15 min**
Timeline introduction and example	**30 min**
Introduction	**10 min**
Timeline exercise	**1 hour**
Feedback and group discussion	**20 min**
The phases of schizophrenia: explanation	**15 min**
Plotting phases on timeline	**15 min**
Introduction to prodromal phase	**15 min**
Identifying prodromal signs exercise	**15 min**
Responses to prodromal signs example and exercise	**30 min**
Acute phase discussion and example	**25 min**
Identification of acute phase symptoms and responses	**20 min**
Remission/recovery phase discussion	**25 min**
Remission/recovery phase exercise	**20 min**
Relapse phase discussion	**15 min**
Relapse phase identification of early warning signs	**20 min**
Cost–benefit analysis of help seeking	**30 min**
Action plan preparation	**25 min**
Living with schizophrenia; review of impact	**45 min**
Future planning exercise	**45 min**

Introduction

The terminology 'person with a diagnosis of schizophrenia' is used in deliberate preference to terms such as 'schizophrenic' or 'patient' to illustrate that the person is much more than their 'illness'. Rather than focus solely on their disorder and its consequences, this module aims to review the person's life in order to look at how their mental health problems have impacted on it, and how to reduce the effects in the future. It is important to focus on the person not just their mental health problems, and to emphasise that life continues despite receiving a diagnosis of schizophrenia. Indeed it may improve once problems are identified and solutions sought.

About me

This exercise is a simple way of exploring a person's personality, likes and dislikes, strengths and weaknesses, and constructs a profile of the person both past and present. Prior to developing mental health problems the person may have lived a 'normal' successful life; they may have been to university, had a career, family, and so on. While the previous statement might be seen as self-evident, because mental health professionals' first contact with the person is often when they are experiencing an acute florid episode, and/or in a psychiatric hospital, it is easy to forget it.

Facilitators should present Handout 1 'What I am like' example sheet. Talk through this example, pointing out the variety of characteristics, likes and dislikes which help to define who we are. Clients should be encouraged to complete Worksheet 1 'What I am like', as fully as possible, with assistance from facilitators as required. Group members then present 'themselves' to the group in turn.

Facilitated group discussion should cover the following five points:

1. People change over time whether or not they have mental health problems.
2. Some characteristics remain the same whether or not a person has mental health problems.
3. Schizophrenia has some influence on a person and their life, but there are also other influences.
4. Previous sources of enjoyment and fulfilment can continue.
5. Nothing stays the same, and future change in oneself and one's lifestyle can be rewarding.

During such a discussion reinforce self-efficacy and self-esteem at any opportunity.

Timeline: my life so far

Constructing a timeline is useful for several reasons. First, it provides a concise and easy way of reviewing one's personal history. Second, it can help to pinpoint significant events and demonstrate how environmental circumstances can influence one's life course. In addition, it illustrates how 'hindsight' can be used to develop an understanding of events and their importance. Timelines can also put into perspective minor crises that might have seemed catastrophic at the time, but with the benefit of 'the long view' can be seen as manageable. Times when a person has coped with adverse life circumstances can also be highlighted to reinforce self-efficacy. Finally, the timeline can be used in later exercises, for example to help in the identification of early signs of the development of psychotic episodes, and to plot identifiable phases of illness and remission.

The timeline exercise takes approximately 1 hour; clients should work individually with assistance from facilitators as required.

An example timeline is presented in Handout 2 'Timeline'. This could be provided as a handout to illustrate the stages of constructing the timeline, alternatively the information could be presented on a flipchart.

A timeline is constructed as follows: provide each person with Worksheet 2 'Timeline'. Ask clients to think back to their earliest memories and significant events and plot them along the line, placing together things that happened at a similar period in time and spacing out along the line events which were more separate in time.

Under each event ask them to write the approximate year it occurred. Events to record include births (of siblings, own children, etc), marriages, deaths, changes in location/house, etc; employment, education, divorce and any other unique or significant events such as special trips, holidays, etc.

Ask clients to add to the line, using a different colour, periods of time in which particular circumstances occurred, for example periods of problematic drinking, drug-taking, physical illness, etc. Finally, with a third colour, ask them to show periods of mental health problems, including hospitalisations, contact with mental health professionals, and so on.

After completing the timelines, clients should feedback to the group. Feedback should include what the person has learnt from their timeline review, what surprised them and any other points of interest.

The phases of schizophrenia

Following on from the timeline exercise, two important concepts can be introduced: prodromes, or the antecedent experiences to a psychotic episode, and the phasic nature of some psychotic disorders.

The following explanation should accompany Handout 3 'The phases of schizophrenia'.

Schizophrenic experiences and their consequences are not stable. They change over time. Although everyone's experiences are different, a general pattern has been observed in people who have been diagnosed as having schizophrenia. Often a 'prodromal' period can be identified before the person experiences any 'psychotic' symptoms such as delusions and hallucinations.

The prodrome is often characterised by a gradual decline in functioning in areas such as work, education, social, interpersonal abilities and personal well-being. This stage can last from between 1 or 2 weeks and several months.

Following this period the 'acute' phase or episode of psychosis occurs. This is characterised by positive symptoms such as delusions and hallucinations. Clinicians sometimes describe people in this stage as having 'florid' symptoms. These experiences are usually treated with antipsychotic medication. It is likely that this stage will pass within weeks or months, and be followed by a period of recovery in which the psychotic symptoms substantially reduce and in some cases disappear completely.

A period of no or few mild symptoms is called 'remission'. With the right treatment, medical, psychological and social, some people can stay in remission for many years. Others experience further 'acute' episodes, usually preceded by relapse prodromal signs or 'early warning signs' that a psychotic episode is likely to be experienced.

Negative symptoms such as lack of motivation and apathy can also fluctuate in severity and show wide individual differences.

Following this explanation group members should be encouraged to plot the probable start of their prodrome on their timeline, together with the start of the first acute episode, the end of the first acute episode, any periods of remission, relapse prodrome and any further acute episodes. Help in delineating such episodes can be given by reviewing medical records and, if available, information from relatives, carers, and so on.

My prodrome: identification and responses

It is often difficult for people to identify and recall the range of experiences they might have had before a noticeable emergence of positive symptoms. Facilitate discussion of the types of problems and experiences which are commonly found in prodromal phases; these are listed in Worksheet 3 'Identification of prodromal signs'. Encourage group members to describe any changes that they noted in themselves in the weeks and months prior to an identified emergence of symptoms. Although the transition from prodromal signs to active symptoms is often not clear, an overlap period might be identified where, for example, a gradual increase in the strength of an unusual belief became problematic.

Distribute Worksheet 3 'Identification of prodromal signs'. This is used to help to identify the onset of mental health decline. Clients should tick any of the signs which they recognise in themselves. Once a number of signs have been identified encourage expansion through discussion, for example 'preoccupation' might be identified and the specifics of this can then be explored.

Clients' responses to their prodromal signs at the time should then be investigated. Responses might include active help-seeking, for example going to the doctor, counsellor or other professional. Responses might also include telling others, such as relatives, friends, colleagues, or indeed keeping the problems to oneself. Self-help or other coping responses should also be elicited, for example relaxation, changes in lifestyle, and so on. Clients might say that they had no response; however, careful examination of the actual response is helpful as it might identify a passive response such as staying in bed or 'trying to carry on as usual'. Responses can also include those of other people, including their attitudes and actions. Handout 4 'Responses to prodromal signs' can be used to aid this process by presenting examples of common responses. Clients should be assisted to complete Worksheet 4 'Responses to prodromal signs' in order to record the important information gathered during this exercise.

Clients should be encouraged to feedback to the group. Facilitate a group discussion of what has been learnt in this session.

My acute phase

There is great variability in the ability of clients to recall the emergence of psychotic symptoms, which might be related to 'insight' as well as to the severity and chronicity of their disorder. Use of information from medical records and relatives can help the client to reconstruct the symptoms, behaviour and consequences of their acute phase. However, the person's own experiences are usually the most meaningful to them.

Psychotic symptoms can appear suddenly or gradually. The development of signs experienced during the prodromal phase might overlap into the acute phase, for example suspiciousness might become paranoia, and therefore it is not always possible to determine the exact start of active psychotic symptoms.

Information about the acute phase can be elicited by simple questions such as 'Following the prodromal phase, what happened next?', 'When did you start to hear voices?', 'Were there any changes over time in their intensity, frequency, effect?', 'When did your thoughts/beliefs start to become problematic?'.

Facilitate discussion using Handout 5 'My acute phase', to present the type of symptoms commonly experienced in the acute phase and typical responses. Using Worksheet 5 'My acute phase', clients should then be encouraged to record the key elements of their acute phase together with their responses to each of these. Responses recorded should be as specific as possible, such as behaviours, emotions. The approximate length of the acute phase should also be recorded. Positive symptoms, such as delusions and hallucinations, will be dealt with more fully in Module 3.

My remission/recovery phase

Following an acute episode where the person experiences hallucinations and/or delusions there is a decline in such symptoms. This is usually assisted by medication. The reduction in symptoms can be absolute or the person may continue to experience residual positive symptoms usually of a lesser frequency, duration or intensity. Residual negative symptoms such as apathy or lack of motivation can also persist. There is often a consequent reduction in the person's ability to function as well as they had previously, for example with regard to work and social abilities. This can be as a direct result of both the process of the disorder and the associated societal responses.

The majority of people undertaking this programme will be in the remission/recovery phase. Each person's stage in recovery will be particular to them. In order to gauge where clients place themselves currently in relation to their previous level of functioning use Worksheet 6 'My recovery phase'. This presents an open-ended list of potential problems, which might include particular positive symptoms, negative symptoms and also general problems related to work and social abilities. The client simply marks their current position on each line from 0 per cent (as bad as it has ever been) to 100 per cent (fully recovered). This provides a simple way of highlighting those areas in which the client feels that they have made progress and those which require further intervention.

My potential relapse phase

Although there are general observable patterns, the course and outcome of psychotic experiences are very variable. Some people will recover completely after one acute episode, others will go on to experience further acute episodes separated by periods of remission, and some will remain more permanently affected, although their symptoms might fluctuate over time.

Relapse should therefore be presented as a possibility rather than as inevitable. Recognition of relapse signs offers the potential for early intervention which might avert relapse and rehospitalisation. If hospitalisation might become necessary early intervention means that this can be planned in advance and in cooperation with the person to avert the damaging effects of forcible sectioning using the Mental Health Act, often when the person is floridly psychotic. Commonly, there is some consistency within an individual in the nature and timing of the early signs of relapse (Herz and Melville, 1980), therefore detailed awareness of one's prodromal signs can act as early warning signs for a potential relapse.

Those who have experienced more than one acute episode should be encouraged to compare the early signs identified prior to each acute episode using Worksheet 3 'Identification of prodromal signs' and Worksheet 4 'Responses to prodromal signs', which can be completed for each episode of relapse. Similarities and differences should be noted, including the nature of any symptoms, time course from identification of the signs to actual relapse, and the response or action taken. Any improved coping abilities or responses should be identified to reinforce the person's self-efficacy. Ideas for action and responses in the event of future episodes should also be discussed.

For those who have not experienced a relapse, the prodromal phase can be reviewed for signs that would serve as good indicators for potential relapse.

The best early warning signs are those that were most obvious to the person or to others. These are usually overt behavioural signs such as spending a lot of time in bed.

Responding to relapse signs

A client's response to early warning signs for relapse is often strongly influenced by their previous experiences of mental health services. Clients might have found difficulty in getting appropriate help, or they might have been misdiagnosed or sectioned against their will. It is not uncommon, therefore, that people do not intend to seek mental health professionals' help in the future. However, such help-seeking can be encouraged by carrying out a cost–benefit analysis of help-seeking. This can identify concerns about informing professionals and also outline the likely consequences of seeking or not seeking help. It can also highlight potential action points to reduce any concerns.

An example of cost–benefit analysis of help-seeking behaviour is presented in Handout 6 'Cost–benefit analysis of seeking professional help'. As a group exercise a cost–benefit analysis can be constructed by drawing it out on a flipchart and asking the group to consider what actions they would take in the case of potential future relapse. Explain that actions and solutions will potentially have both good and bad consequences, and both long- and short-term consequences. To make a good decision these consequences need to be weighed up and a judgement made. Complete the four sections of the chart; start with the short-term gains followed by long-term gains and then move on to short-term costs and finally long-term costs. Following this the group should be asked to decide whether seeking professional help is a preferred option. As the points are raised, concerns should be addressed; for example, if concerns are expressed about attending their general practitioner, discuss whether this is an accurate perception, perhaps by using evidence from previous contacts. If there is a potential problem, this can be 'problem solved', for example by addressing whether it would be useful to change GP, whether it would help to go with a friend, and so on. It is also worth stressing that previous negative experiences, such as difficulty being believed or taken seriously, are far less likely now that a formal diagnosis has been made. Building a good relationship with mental health professionals, such as CPNs, social workers, psychologists, and so on, also improves the chances of a more favourable outcome should relapse occur; for example, through being able to discuss choices and preferred options well in advance of an acute episode.

The cost–benefit analysis exercise will have demonstrated that seeking help is a positive option. In order to formalise this, individual action plans should be created which detail how to seek help. These should be clear and simple and contain the information that each client requires, including names and telephone numbers as appropriate. Help clients to complete Worksheet 7 'Early warning signs action plan'. Ensure that each client knows who to contact, for example their doctor, social worker, psychologist or other key worker; how contact should be made depending on the circumstances, for example by telephone or appointment. Discuss when and what to report and set thresholds depending on significance of the problem and imminence of potential relapse, for example a sleep disturbance might not be problematic if it lasts for one or two nights but might become significant after a week depending on the person's previous history.

Living with schizophrenia: reducing the impact

The final section of this module focuses on enabling the person to examine the aspects of their lives which they would like to improve. This might entail giving up bad habits, modifying previous life goals, for example regarding their career, reducing demands that make life stressful, deciding on new attainable goals and looking at new challenges. Three worksheets completed earlier in the module can be used to collate useful information: Worksheet 1 'What I am like', Worksheet 2 'Timeline' and Worksheet 6 'My recovery phase'. Using the timeline to explore 'good times' and 'bad times' can help to highlight areas which the person might want to change. These might include maladaptive coping strategies, as well as areas which might be developed to improve quality of life. Similarly, the completed exercise: 'What I am like' can be reviewed and the information used to help identify areas of future development, together with items identified as current or ongoing problems from examination of the recovery phase.

This information can be brought together to complete Worksheet 8 'Future me', which is a guide to exploring types of changes that could reduce the impact of living with a diagnosis of schizophrenia. If this is carried out as a group exercise each person can present their ideas, and group members can be encouraged to offer their advice and suggestions to each other.

What I am like: example

	Past	Present
My character/ personality	*Sensitive* *Energetic* *Creative* *Independent*	*Quiet* *Thoughtful* *A good listener* *Creative* *Resilient*
My hobbies/interests	*Cycling* *Running* *Astronomy* *Buddhism*	*Reading* *Computers* *Collecting fossils* *Buddhism* *Singing*
People close to me	*Mother* *Sister* *School friend* *Partner*	*Sister* *Friend (Jo)* *Friend (Liz)*
What I am good at	*PE (school)* *Maths* *Singing*	*Computers* *Making things* *Singing*
Employment	*Shop assistant* *Post Office*	*Hospital shop*
Dislikes	*Spiders* *Sprouts* *Arguments*	*Spiders* *Noise* *Untidiness*
Likes	*Jokes* *Chocolate* *Animals*	*Jokes* *Sunday roast* *Time on my own* *Day trips*
What I would like to do in the future		*Learn to play the guitar* *Join a choir* *Get a part-time job* *Live near the sea*

What I am like

	Past	Present
My character/ personality		
My hobbies/interests		
People close to me		
What I am good at		
Employment		
Dislikes		
Likes		
What I would like to do in the future		

Timeline: example

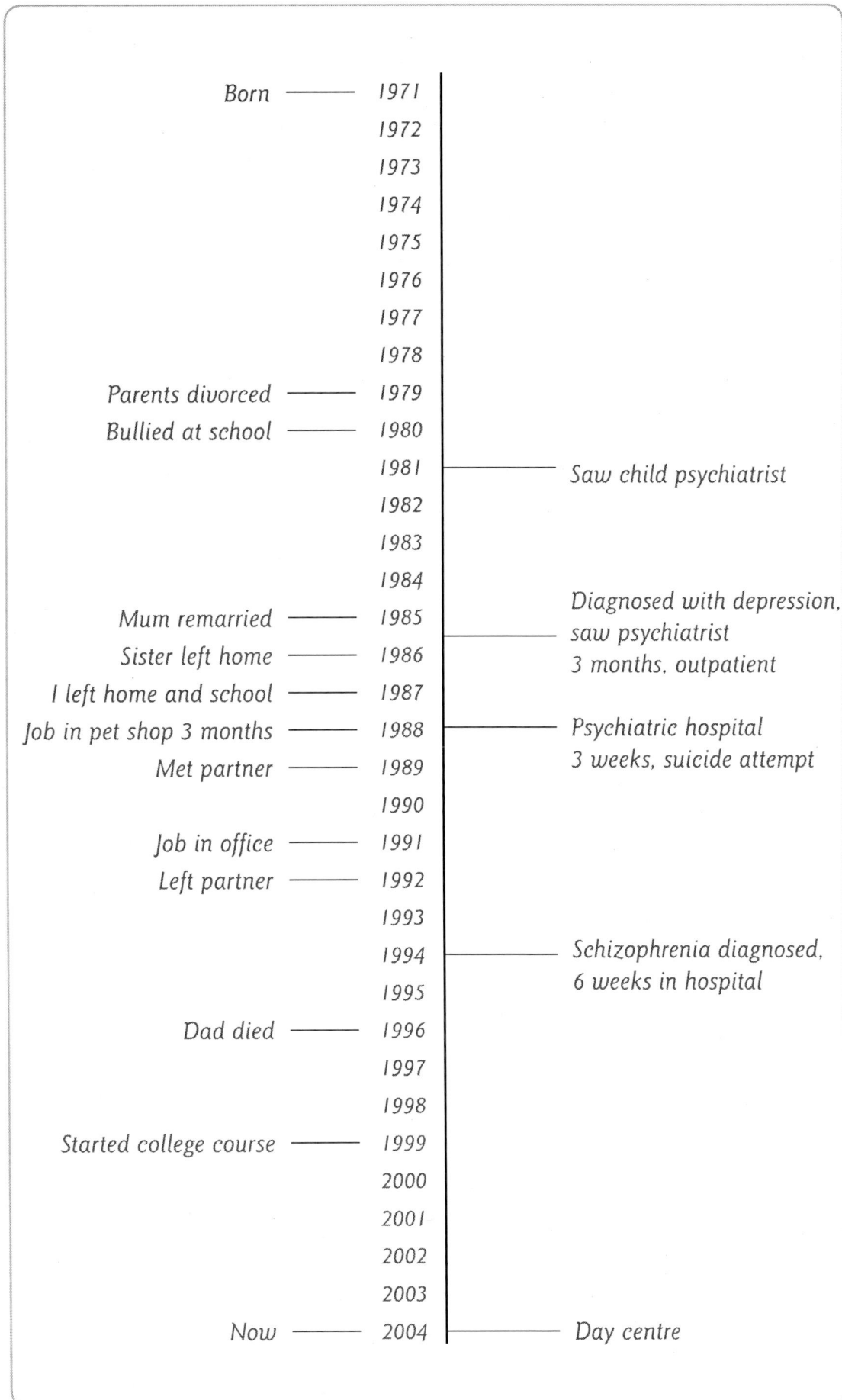

Born	1971	
	1972	
	1973	
	1974	
	1975	
	1976	
	1977	
	1978	
Parents divorced	1979	
Bullied at school	1980	
	1981	Saw child psychiatrist
	1982	
	1983	
	1984	
Mum remarried	1985	Diagnosed with depression, saw psychiatrist 3 months, outpatient
Sister left home	1986	
I left home and school	1987	
Job in pet shop 3 months	1988	Psychiatric hospital 3 weeks, suicide attempt
Met partner	1989	
	1990	
Job in office	1991	
Left partner	1992	
	1993	
	1994	Schizophrenia diagnosed, 6 weeks in hospital
	1995	
Dad died	1996	
	1997	
	1998	
Started college course	1999	
	2000	
	2001	
	2002	
	2003	
Now	2004	Day centre

MODULE 2

Timeline

The phases of schizophrenia

Prodrome	Acute	Remission/ recovery	Relapse Prodrome
For example: Reduced social contact Fear of 'going mad' Loss of interest	Delusions Hallucinations 'Positive' symptoms	Reduction or loss of symptoms Some residual difficulties	Early warning signs of possible impending acute phase

Each of the phases can last for weeks or months.

Identification of prodromal signs

Prodromal sign	This happened to me (✓)
I thought I was going 'mad' or going to have a nervous breakdown	
I lost interest in things	
I became more emotional	
I could not concentrate	
I became preoccupied with things	
I felt I did not 'fit in'	
I thought something bad was going to happen	
I felt overwhelmed	
I did not look after myself (eg diet, appearance)	
I had no energy	
I felt confused	
I thought I was losing control of myself	
I was bored	
I had lots of new thoughts	
I could not make decisions	
I thought people did not understand me	
I felt lonely	
I had bad dreams	
I wanted to be on my own	
I was not interested in sex	
I felt frightened	
I felt very energetic	
My sex drive increased	
I felt unreal	
I was more interested in religious ideas	
I felt excited	
I could not sleep	
I felt angry	
I became aggressive	
Other (please state)	

Responses to prodromal signs: example

My prodromal signs	My responses
I felt overwhelmed	*I could not cope with work and started taking time off, going in late, etc*
I could not make decisions	*I did less because I spent so long thinking about what might happen*
I was not interested in sex	*My partner got angry and fed up with me. We stopped talking*
I felt unreal	*I did not tell anyone how I felt because I could not describe it and thought they would not understand*
I felt angry	*I shouted at people and felt irritated by them*

MODULE 2

Responses to prodromal signs

My prodromal signs	My responses

My acute phase: example

My acute phase Approximate time scale = **6 weeks**	Response
I felt suspicious of people and concerned that I could be harmed	*Avoided people*
I thought people could hear my thoughts	*Avoided people*
I thought the telephone was bugged	*I did not telephone people* *I disconnected the telephone*
I thought the television news was about me	*I smashed the TV. My mum phoned the doctor. I was admitted to hospital*
I felt panicky and scared	*I was prescribed medication*

My acute phase

My acute phase Approximate time scale =	Response

My recovery phase

Mark each line to show where you are in terms of recovery, compared with how you were before you were 'ill':

- 'Positive' symptoms (specify), for example voices

0% 25% 50% 75% 100%

- 'Negative' symptoms (specify), for example apathy

0% 25% 50% 75% 100%

- Ability to work

0% 25% 50% 75% 100%

- Social interaction

0% 25% 50% 75% 100%

- General 'well-being'

0% 25% 50% 75% 100%

Cost–benefit analysis of seeking professional help

	Benefits	Costs
Short-term	Feel relief Feel less scared	Have to make appointment with GP who does not like me Might have to go to hospital
Long-term	Get the right help Get better sooner! Spend less time in hospital Learn more about my problems and how to cope Find people to talk to about my problems Meeting people with the same experiences	Stigma of 'mental illness'

Early warning signs action plan

Who to contact

How to contact

When to report

What to report

Future me (page 1 of 2)

Thinking about the future, complete this sheet to identify your goals for the next year:

- Reducing demands
  What would make your life less stressful?

- List some things that you have enjoyed that you might like to 'get back into', for example hobbies, interests

- Breaking bad habits
  What would you like to stop doing? For example drinking, smoking

Future me (page 2 of 2)

- Changing direction, for example work, relationships

- Things to work on; set yourself some targets, for example exercise, diet, friendships

- New horizons, for example goals, aspirations, ambitions

MODULE 3

Understanding and managing positive symptoms

The fact that patients diagnosed as 'schizophrenic' have a circumscribed set of irrational beliefs does not mean that they are irrational individuals.

(Aaron Beck, 1994)

Overview of Module

- Introduction
- Levels of intervention for positive symptoms
- Level 1: Identification, assessment and monitoring of positive symptoms
- Level 2: Reducing associated distress, coping strategy enhancement and behavioural symptom management
- Level 3: Psycho-education, psychological models, introducing doubt
- Level 4: Peripheral challenging
- Level 5: Modification of symptoms
- Level 6: Schema-focused interventions

Suggested Session Plans

Module 3 includes interventions which should be carried out in individual one-to-one sessions. Time allocations for such interventions are provided as a guide to planning these sessions.

Level 1	
Identification of precipitating factors to auditory hallucinations and construction of monitoring record	**20 min**
Personal questionnaire construction	**30 min**
Beliefs About Voices Questionnaire (BAVQ)	**15 min**
Diary sheet construction	**15 min**
Level 2	
Coping strategies for positive symptoms	**35 min**
Coping strategy enhancement behavioural analysis	**35 min**
Coping strategy enhancement case example	**20 min**
Level 3	
Hallucinations as information processing errors guided learning	**1 hour**
Additional coping strategies and discussion	**30 min**
Relationship between thoughts, feelings and behaviour and exercise	**30 min**
Ten ways we get things wrong	**40 min**
Thinking errors	**20 min**
Level 4	
Examining belief exercise	**45 min**
Improving judgements and discussion	**45 min**
Level 5	
Introduction to objective examination	**20 min**
Case example exercise	**30 min**
Individual supplementary intervention	**45 min**
Behavioural experiment technique	**20 min**
Behavioural experiment case example	**20 min**
Individual supplementary intervention	**45 min**
Level 6	
Individual intervention	
Prejudice exercise	**45 min**
Own belief exercise	**45 min**
Leading to schema-focused interventions as appropriate	

Introduction

A diagnosis of schizophrenia is made on the basis of symptoms, primarily the identification of positive symptoms classified as hallucinations and delusions. Psychiatry promotes the concept of these symptoms as bizarre phenomena that are entirely divorced from normal thought and sensory processes. They are seen as the essence of 'madness'. This assumption can lead people with a diagnosis of schizophrenia to feel abnormal, scared and ashamed of their symptoms and as a consequence less likely to talk to others about such symptoms.

This module aims to:

1 Promote a better understanding of delusions and hallucinations. To destigmatise and demystify them in order to reduce associated distress.
2 Present a psychological understanding of why hallucinations and delusions might occur.
3 Help people to develop coping strategies for problematic symptoms.

Levels of intervention for positive symptoms

When working with people's positive symptoms, the most appropriate type of intervention will be determined by the person's specific goals and their preferred coping style, which may change over time. For example, some people prefer to view their symptoms as pathological, distinct and separate from themselves. This might lead to a strong reluctance to examine them in any way, and instead the goal might be to cope with the associated distress and relieve the symptoms by medication. Other people prefer to 'integrate' the experience into their lives and develop an understanding of the experiences in order to normalise them. In this circumstance it would be appropriate to examine the misinterpretations and thinking errors, and analyse the formation of delusional beliefs. In some instances particular delusional beliefs can engender positive feelings as well as negative ones, such as feeling special, chosen or powerful. In these circumstances it is necessary to gauge whether modification of the delusion would result in a better quality of life for the person or would remove a powerful source of self-identity, which is not significantly interfering with their life. It is important to ensure that deconstructing a delusional belief is not likely to have negative consequences, and it is important to explore the likely consequences of relinquishing particular beliefs before deciding whether such interventions are appropriate.

A good collaborative, therapeutic relationship is the key to gauging the most productive type of intervention. The different levels of intervention can be summarised as follows:

1 Identification, assessment and monitoring of positive symptoms.
2 Reducing associated distress, coping strategy enhancement and behavioural symptom management.
3 Psycho-education, psychological models, introducing doubt.
4 Peripheral challenging: 'what if?' hypothetical contradiction.
5 Modification of symptoms, examining, questioning and alternative explanations.
6 Schema-focused interventions.

The level of intervention at which to start addressing positive symptoms is dependent on the client's individual knowledge, understanding and readiness.

Level 1: Identification, assessment and monitoring of positive symptoms

Ideally, the assessment of positive symptoms should meet three criteria: be tailored to the individual; be simple rather than complex; and be purposeful rather than an end in itself. Formal assessment measures of positive symptoms were outlined in Part II: Assessment. Assessment can be used as an intervention in that it can increase awareness and knowledge of one's symptoms, indicate precipitants to symptoms, fluctuations over time and areas for potential direct intervention.

Identification of precipitating factors to auditory hallucinations

In a study of coping mechanisms for persistent auditory hallucinations, it was found that the best outcome was associated with using a limited number of strategies consistently 'particularly when the patient was aware of environmental precipitants' (Falloon and Talbot, 1981).

Explain to the group that keeping a record of experiences of hallucinations can help to identify precipitants to hallucinations and thus to suggest possible interventions to reduce or cope with such experiences (Slade, 1971). Two types of variable are commonly found to precipitate hallucinations: mood state, which might include tension, sadness, difficulty concentrating, anger; and environmental variables, which might include noise level, number of people, activity level. Assist clients to devise their own monitoring record to help identify any precipitating factors. What to include on such a record form should be decided in collaboration with the client. Common environmental and mood state precipitants are given in Handout 1 'Common environmental and mood state precipitants' and a sample hallucination monitoring record is presented in Worksheet 1 'Hallucination monitoring record'. The client should be encouraged to complete records three times each day, morning, afternoon and evening, for a period of two weeks. The ratings of environmental and mood state variables can then be compared to look for differences between when the hallucination was 'present' and 'absent'. Any significant differences will indicate likely precipitants.

Analysis of individual records is likely to indicate potential interventions; for example, if voices are more likely to be heard in situations of high tension and anxiety and in the absence of people, it would follow that coping strategies might include learning techniques to reduce anxiety and seeking out social interaction.

Monitoring symptoms with personal questionnaires

Personal questionnaires enable the specific characteristics of a symptom to be assessed and monitored. They have been used primarily with delusions, but can be modified to provide informative data for many psychotic symptoms. Personal questionnaires can be constructed using any of the characteristics which appear to be relevant to the individual. In this way specific tailored questionnaires can be constructed, and different questionnaires can also be constructed for the same individual to monitor different symptoms. Questionnaires can be completed at a frequency appropriate to monitor change specific to the person. This might be daily, weekly or monthly, or prior to and following specific interventions. Any of the following measurable characteristics of delusions can be used for constructing personal questionnaires:

- Conviction: the certainty with which the delusion is held.
- Importance: how important the delusion is to the person.
- Preoccupation: the pervasiveness of the delusion, for example the percentage of time each day that is spent ruminating about delusional concerns.
- Distress: the associated negative feelings, for example anxiety, anger.
- Coping: how well the person feels they manage the delusional belief and its consequences.

- Perspective: the person's awareness of how others will view their delusion.
- Action: specific behaviours likely to result in delusion, for example checking, avoidance.

The characteristics can be measured by the most appropriate method, for example by using percentage ratings or a simple Likert scale. Examples of personal questionnaires are shown in Handout 2 'Personal questionnaire example 1' and Handout 3 'Personal questionnaire example 2'.

Construction of personal questionnaires should be done on an individual basis. Explain the rationale for personal questionnaires and design the questionnaire with the client, tailoring it to their individual needs. In particular consider the nature, content and frequency of the symptoms.

Detailed assessment of auditory hallucinations

If cognitive intervention is indicated specific assessment of the person's understanding of and responses to their auditory hallucinations can be undertaken using the *Beliefs About Voices Questionnaire*, BAVQ (Chadwick and Birchwood, 1995). This self-report instrument measures 'malevolence of voices', for example 'my voice is punishing me for something I have done', as well as benevolence, for example 'my voice wants to help me'. It also measures engagement, for example whether the person listens to and courts their voices, and resistance, for example whether the person tells their voice to go away. Research using this questionnaire found, perhaps not surprisingly, that voices perceived to be malevolent were resisted, whereas those perceived to be benevolent were courted. This scale can help to identify areas for cognitive therapy and other interventions, and can also indicate hallucinations which the patient does not wish to change.

Diaries can be a very helpful way to gather information about and monitor specific symptoms. Simple diaries such as shown in Worksheet 2 'Diary sheet for monitoring symptoms' can be used to look for fluctuations in symptoms, patterns, coping abilities, precipitants and consequences.

Level 2: Reducing associated distress, coping strategy enhancement and behavioural symptom management

A study of the ways in which people cope with their symptoms of schizophrenia found a variety of techniques that could be categorised as behaviour change, socialisation, cognitive control, use of medical care and behaviours which were likely to have been identified by others as symptomatic of the illness (Carr, 1988). Just as people adapt to other chronic illnesses, many people with a diagnosis of schizophrenia find ways of reducing the impact of their symptoms.

Groupwork with people with a diagnosis of schizophrenia is particularly productive when generating ideas and sharing experiences about how to cope. Sessions to explore individuals' current and previous coping strategies can gather together methods and techniques that clients have found to be useful in the management of their symptoms. This reinforces self-efficacy and promotes the idea of being involved and creative in managing one's symptoms.

Facilitate a brainstorming exercise by asking the group members how they cope with positive symptoms. This will produce a number of different ways of coping with delusions and hallucinations such as those listed in Handout 4 'How we cope with positive symptoms'. The list generated could be transferred into a handout for the group. Once a list has been produced the facilitators should lead a guided discussion of these coping strategies by grouping them into categories, as shown in Handout 5 'Categories of coping strategies'.

This procedure demonstrates that there is a wide range of techniques that can be used to cope with symptoms.

Maladaptive or problematic coping strategies might be elicited, such as drinking alcohol or shouting. The appropriateness, usefulness and potential problems arising from such actions should be discussed by examining the short- and long-term costs and benefits of such strategies. Alternative techniques could be discussed, particularly those within the same category, which might provide non-problematic options. For example, a client whose interpersonal relationships were seriously affected by his shouting at voices found that he could produce the same relief from the voices, while not becoming alienated from others, by singing.

Coping strategy enhancement or CSE involves a behavioural analysis of psychotic symptoms and the person's coping strategies, which informs training and practice in specified coping methods (Tarrier, 1992). Once clients have identified strategies that they have found to be useful or might wish to try, these can be examined in more detail. The effectiveness of each strategy can be discussed to gain information on (a) how effective the strategy is, for example: negligible, moderate or very effective; (b) how consistently the strategy is used and reasons for non-use; and (c) if coping strategies have variable success, elicit under which conditions this variability occurs. Facilitators can guide discussion with each group member to elicit and decide on the person's 'top' strategies, which are most likely to be effective. The next step is to try to maximise the person's chances of success with the strategy by ensuring its consistent and systematic use. This can be done by agreeing the following:

- The exact detail of when, how and where the strategy will be used
- Discuss any obstacles to use of the strategy and agree solutions, for example, supplementary coping strategies
- Practise the strategy with the facilitator, if appropriate
- Practise the strategy in imagination, if appropriate
- Practise the strategy between sessions and record outcome on a monitoring form
- Review the record and implementation of coping strategy at each session and reinforce its continued use, discussing any problems arising and generate solutions
- If necessary, the coping strategy can be modified or an alternative strategy selected.

This detailed and structured approach may appear to be overly prescriptive; however, giving brief and general advice is seldom sufficient. As with most psychological interventions, consistency and systematic use are vital for maximising successful outcomes. Facilitators should present the coping strategy enhancement case example to illustrate how CSE works in practice.

Coping strategy enhancement: case example

Case example

SARAH is a 24-year-old woman with relatively persistent auditory hallucinations of a critical and judgemental nature. Her chosen coping strategy was one of direct action, telling the voices to go away.

- Effectiveness checklist
  (a) How effective is the strategy? Moderate
  (b) How consistently is the strategy used? 50–60%
- Reasons for non-use
  If people are around, I use it less. If I have to concentrate on something else, for example, computer lesson, I don't use it.

- When most successful? On my own when I feel calm, when I feel strong. When least successful? If tired, if feeling depressed.
- Agreeing the detail
  (a) When to use strategy: every time I hear the voices, usually four to five times a day.
  (b) How to use the strategy: repetitive phrases are best, especially if spoken quietly in a calm voice.

Sarah developed the notion of a 'calming mantra' and compiled a phrase, to repeat directing the voices to go away.

- Obstacles
  (a) Need to be alone. Possible solutions: actively seek solitude when appropriate, for example when in television lounge find an excuse for leaving temporarily.
  (b) Is difficult to use when feeling tired or anxious. Possible solutions: use my relaxation tape, try the technique, it might make me feel calmer.
- Practice strategy
  In individual session with facilitator.
- Record form (extract)

Day	Time	Location	Used strategy (tick or cross)	Rate outcome Success 1–10
Monday	11.15 am	Out walking on own	✔	5
Monday	12.30 pm	Dining room	✗	1
Monday	7.30 pm	TV lounge	✔	6

Through coping strategy modification, after 6 weeks: a good level of effective use was achieved. Sarah then managed to develop her calming mantra technique so that she could use this effectively 'in her head' rather than speaking it aloud, which increased the variety of situations in which it could be used.

Level 3: Psycho-education, psychological models, introducing doubt

This level of intervention encourages clients to examine alternative ways of looking at their beliefs, thoughts, delusions and hallucinations. There is no direct challenge or modification of symptoms but the concept of doubt rather than certainty in one's beliefs and perceptions is introduced.

Hallucinations as information-processing errors

There are several theories as to what causes hallucinations, for example biochemical imbalance, neuroanatomical abnormalities. However, there is no consensus about the aetiology of hallucinations. Although little is known about the neurophysiology of auditory and visual hallucinations, it is possible to offer an explanation of mistakes, to which we are all susceptible, as a way of demonstrating that not all of our perceptions are accurate.

Facilitators should present a brief explanation of perceptual errors as follows.

Information comes to us via our senses: hearing, seeing, touching, smelling and tasting. Commonly people assume that our senses are a purely mechanical process but in fact they are strongly influenced by psychological processes. Just as the brain is not merely a computer, the eye is not a camera and the ear is not a radio receiver. Our senses provide our brains with information, which is encoded using electrical impulses via patterns of neural activity to represent the world around us. Perception is not only determined by the stimulus patterns, it is a dynamic searching for the best interpretation of the available data. Perception is strongly influenced by our previous knowledge and experience. Our senses do not give us a picture of the world directly: they provide evidence and a checking of ideas about what is there.

This idea can be illustrated by showing clients pictures of 'ambiguous figures', a good source of such examples is *Eye and Brain, the Psychology of Seeing* (Gregory, 1979). Ambiguous figures can be drawn on a flipchart as shown in Figure 2. Ask group members what they see; some will see profiles of two faces, others will see a vase. This is dependent on whether they interpret the black image as foreground or background, and illustrates how the same pattern of stimulation to the eye can give rise to different perceptions. Perception of objects is more than sensory input.

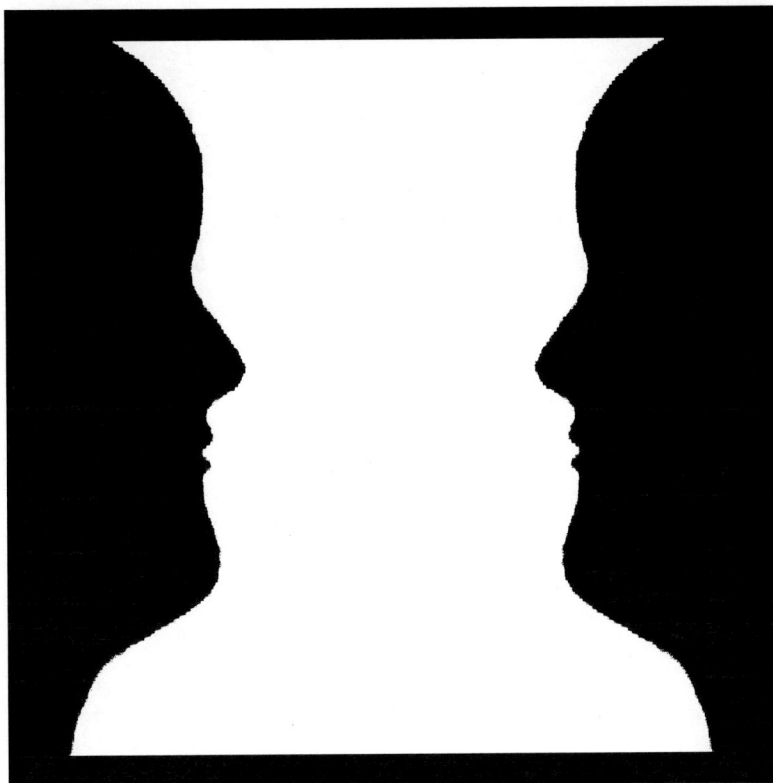

Figure 2 Figure/ground Ambiguous figure

This is also the case for auditory information. Explain that we all selectively attend to and organise the information provided by our senses. Give an example of being at a crowded party where it is possible to switch attention from one conversation to another. Each time the new conversation stands out, becomes the foreground, the others become indistinct background noise.

This can be further illustrated by playing a piece of music; it is best to choose a piece which has two or more simultaneous melodic lines, for example Mozart, Beethoven or Bach. Ask group members to attend to one theme and to follow it. After a few minutes, stop and replay the same piece. This time clients should attend to a different theme. Stop and replay the music for a third time, instructing clients to follow one instrument, for example flute or violin only. Lead a group discussion of people's experiences of this exercise to bring out the following points:

- Some people find it easier than others to follow one theme or instrument. This can be influenced by past experience.
- We can learn to follow the pattern from instrument to instrument.
- As the same piece is listened to repeatedly, we hear new themes.

- The theme attended to is the figure, everything else becomes ground.
- The variety of possible themes and instruments is not obvious until you begin to attend to them.
- Once a particular way of organising the music is found, it is easier to hear and to anticipate the next phrases.

The above exercise illustrates how perceptual experiences are influenced by the individual's way of organising, classifying and interpreting sensory messages.

Thinking is influenced by several basic components: sensory processes, perception, attention, pattern recognition, memory and language. We therefore need a sophisticated processing system in order to help us use this information. It is likely that we have several different processes, which can work independently but are monitored by a 'supervisory' process. One result of the complex nature of human information processing is that we can have different states of awareness. For example, when we become engrossed in a book or play our awareness of the real environment around us is suppressed. Similarly, we can become 'lost in thought' or daydream where we enter a trance-like state. Meditation can produce special states of focused awareness. Other examples of altered states of awareness include states induced by fatigue, high emotions, drugs and alcohol.

Auditory, tactile, olfactory and visual hallucinations often occur when people are very tired, aroused, under stress, deprived of sleep or food, or under the influence of drugs. Considering the wide variety of possible experiences, and the abilities we have for generating fantasies and imagined experiences, it is understandable that sometimes our mind 'plays tricks' and we are misled by hallucinatory experiences.

Ask group members if they have ever experienced mental states such as déjà vu (already seen), the state of feeling that we have previously experienced some current event; or 'jamais vu' (never seen), when a present experience seems to be a novel one even if it really is a familiar event that one has encountered many times before. Explain that these altered states are common experiences. These experiences, like hallucinations, are likely to be caused by confusion in our 'supervisory' information processing system. This system has to work out situations by using information from past experiences together with that arriving at the sensory systems. The system sometimes confuses newly arriving information with that provided by the memory system. When perceptions that are really based on information from the memory and imagination are thought to have come from information provided by the sensory systems, the present experience is hallucinatory.

Ensure that enough time is available at the end of this explanation for further discussion and clarification as needed. Group members should also be encouraged to describe their personal hallucinatory experiences, if appropriate.

For further reading on this subject see *Human Information Processing* (Lindsay and Norman, 1977).

Facilitate a group discussion to elicit coping strategies relevant to this understanding of hallucinations as information-processing errors. Strategies might include checking out whether the person feels exhausted or other possible precursors to information processing errors. Distribute Handout 6 'More coping strategies for hallucinations', to guide further discussion.

Thinking errors, misperceptions and delusions

Introduce the concept that our thoughts always mediate between a situation and our responses to that situation. This is presented in Figure 3, which shows a simple model of the relationship between thoughts, feelings and behaviour. The following exercise can be used to illustrate this relationship. Prepare a flipchart with three columns headed 'Thoughts', 'Feelings', 'Behaviour', and present the following scenario.

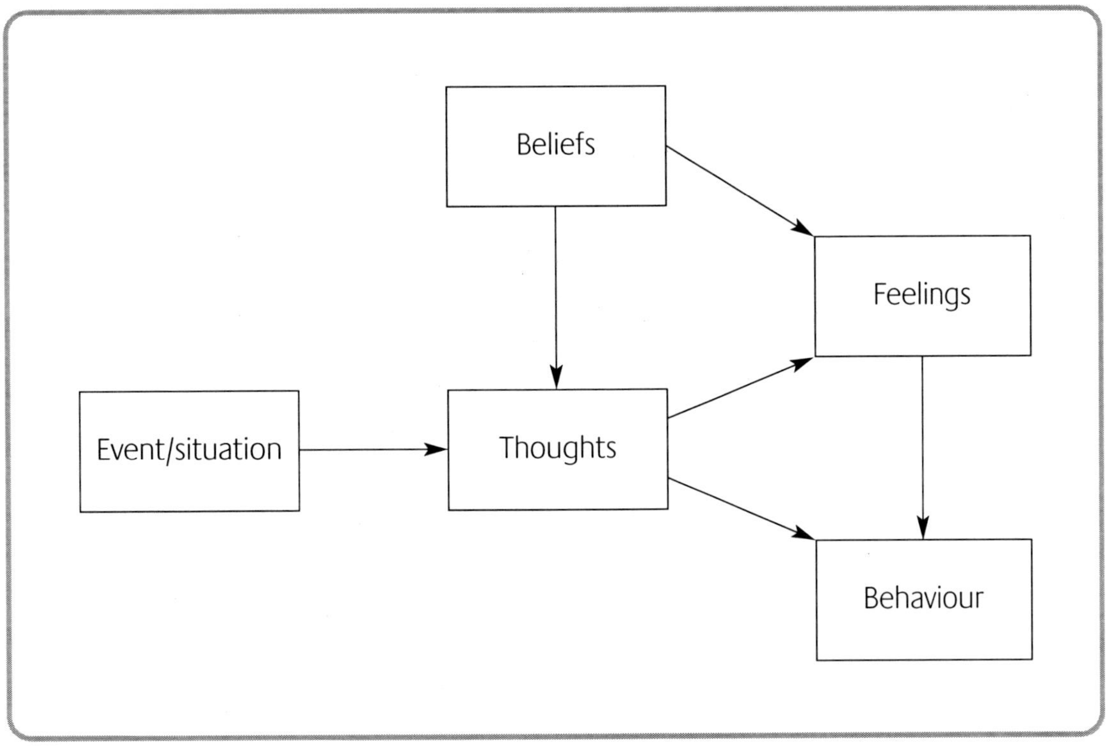

Figure 3 Simple model of the relationship between thoughts, feelings and behaviour

> You are alone in your house, it is late at night, and you are asleep. Suddenly you are awakened by a noise downstairs. What do you *think*?

The responses to this should be listed on the flipchart in the 'Thoughts' column. Elicit only thoughts at this stage. Second, ask each group member, having had that particular thought, how it would make them *feel*. List this on the flipchart in the 'Feelings' column. Third, ask what they would *do* in response to the thought and list this under 'Behaviour'. An example of likely responses is presented in Table 1 to illustrate the link between thoughts, feelings and behaviour.

Thought	Feelings	Behaviour
It's a burglar	Angry/scared	Get up and investigate
It's the cat	Annoyed	Go and let it in
It's the central heating	Mild irritation	Turn over and go back to sleep
It's a ghost	Scared	Hide under the bed covers

Table 1 Example to illustrate link between thoughts, feelings and behaviour

This exercise illustrates that it is not the event itself that causes us to behave in certain ways, but the way in which we think about or interpret the situation. Our thoughts or cognitions always intervene between an event and our response to that event. Our thoughts are influenced by previous experience and our underlying beliefs.

Facilitators should lead a discussion to explore the following points.

Most people consider that what they think is accurate. Similarly, most people assume that their beliefs are true. In reality thoughts and beliefs can be distorted in a number of ways. We do not process information in the same way as computers. The way we gather and use information is complex and is dependent on our physiological, chemical, biological, social, environmental and psychological circumstances. Our thoughts and beliefs are specific to us and our personal constructions of reality are to a greater or lesser extent inaccurate.

Distribute copies of Handout 7, 'Ten ways we get things wrong'. A discussion should be facilitated for each of the ten ways in which common biases and inaccuracies occur. Facilitators should draw out examples from group members, and provide personal examples where appropriate. Point 10, 'Thinking errors' is particularly important and should be elaborated by detailing eight common thinking errors, as described in Handout 8 'Common thinking errors'. Following this exercise introduce the idea of delusions as cognitive mistakes that are selectively reinforced, for example by superstitious thinking, judgement bias, etc. Rather than viewing delusional beliefs as fixed pathological phenomena, this introduces the idea that the belief might be false as many of our beliefs might be. 'Delusional beliefs are not categorically different to over-valued ideas or normal beliefs but are at the extreme end of the continuum of consensual agreement', (Turkington et al, 1996). Such beliefs are held despite evidence to the contrary as are many of our beliefs. However, this way of conceptualising delusions suggests that they might be amenable to change if contrary evidence is examined in this context.

In summary, there is no right or wrong way to view a situation. Our judgements inform our beliefs and opinions. They are subject to influences which undermine to a greater or lesser extent the accuracy of those judgements.

Level 4: Peripheral challenging

This level of intervention does not directly challenge individuals' own beliefs but teaches techniques for challenging by using example vignettes.

Examining beliefs exercise

This exercise illustrates how factors such as selective attention, misjudgements and thinking errors can create and reinforce 'delusional beliefs'. The exercise also provides an opportunity to use basic techniques in order to explore the accuracy of beliefs. Present the vignette described in Handout 9 'Examining beliefs vignette: Bill'. After reading through the vignette, ask group members to answer the following questions:

1. How likely is it that Bill's belief is true? Write down your initial rating: 0 = Not at all, 10 = Definitely true.
2. What evidence does Bill use to arrive at his conclusion? Answers should be listed on the flipchart. Likely answers include:
   - illegal drugs found at Heathrow
   - drugs came from Jamaica
   - Jamie's father is based at Heathrow
   - Jamie's father flies to Jamaica
   - Jamie's father has a lot of money, sports car, house with swimming pool

- Sam is looking pale and sweaty
- Sam spends time at Jamie's and isolating self in bedroom
- Sam wearing long-sleeve T-shirt, perhaps to hide needle marks
- Sam sullen, moody, facial acne.

3 What are the alternative explanations for Sam's behaviour? List answers on the flipchart. Likely responses include:
- Pale and sweaty: this might have been due to being out training for triathlon
- Time in bedroom, sullen, moody, facial acne: this is typical of teenagers' behaviour
- Long-sleeved football shirt: possibly a favourite top, becoming conscious of what he wears, no longer likes his mother's taste in clothing
- Spending time at Jamie's: could be using swimming pool to train for triathlon.

4 What contrary evidence is Bill not considering? List responses on flipchart. Responses might include:
- Sam has been selected for country triathlon event: must be very fit, good stamina, unlikely if injecting heroin
- If Jamie's father is a drug trafficker, involved in million pound drug deals, he would not be interested in getting his son's school friend hooked
- Airline pilots are not usually involved in drug trafficking
- There is no evidence from school that Sam is absent or his schoolwork is poor.

5 What thinking errors and misjudgements might Bill be making? List answers on the flipchart. Answers likely to include:
- Jumping to conclusions, 2 + 2 = 5 thinking. There are no direct links between Jamie's father and drug trafficking. There are only vague coincidences, such as he works at Heathrow airport
- Selective attention: Jamie's father flies to Jamaica: this is a popular holiday destination. He also flies to 22 other destinations
- Ignoring contradictory evidence, see above
- Ignoring alternative explanations, for example he is assuming that the money comes from drug trafficking, however, airline pilots are relatively well paid, it is possible that his wife also has a well-paid job, he might have inherited money, etc.

6 Ask group members to write down their considered rating of how likely it is that Bill's belief is true, 0 = Not at all, 10 = Definitely true. Discuss any changes in initial and considered ratings.

Improving judgements

Inform group members that there are many ways of avoiding errors of judgement. There are a number of questions which we can ask ourselves to improve our accuracy.

Provide clients with Handout 10 'How to improve judgements'. Go through each point in turn, leading a discussion on how to use these methods and any obstacles to this which might be raised.

It is possible that some clients will wish to examine their own delusional beliefs; this opportunity should be provided when they are ready to do so. This should be decided on an individual basis in full collaboration with the client. Further work on objective examination of beliefs is provided in the next level of intervention.

Level 5: Modification of symptoms

This level of intervention aims to directly modify symptoms. The two main methods are objective examination and behavioural experiments.

Objective examination

Objective examination does not involve contradicting the person's beliefs. The core of the delusion is not questioned, and this ensures that a collaborative and non-threatening approach can be pursued. The beliefs are rather 'checked out' by the person themselves with guidance from the facilitator. The analogy of being a scientist setting up an experiment to test a hypothesis or a detective examining all aspects of a case, can be used to describe how the person can become an objective examiner of their own beliefs.

The scientist or detective might have some preconceived ideas, strong suspicions, or hunches regarding their enquiry. However, they need to consider all the evidence to be objective and open minded in examining their hypotheses.

Facilitators can guide a discussion on how a scientist/detective would go about their task. Ideas generated could be discussed in relation to how they would help in remaining objective. Examples might include:

- Discussion with colleagues
- Not working in isolation
- Generating alternative hypotheses: 'what if?' scenarios

- Using a variety of sources of information
- Seeking independent expert advice
- Being able to distinguish facts from opinions
- Asking questions.

This discussion should lead on to how group members can be objective in examining their own beliefs by asking the right questions. This builds on the ideas in Level 4 on how to improve judgements. The example case vignette of Jane should be used to explore the technique; this is provided in Handout 11 'Case vignette: Jane'. After reading out this vignette, facilitators should follow the objective examination questions, write up each question in turn and elicit likely answers from members before giving the actual case answers. The questions and typical answers are provided in Handout 12 'Objective examination of belief: Jane'.

Clients should be encouraged to examine their own beliefs in this way. This should be done during individual sessions with their therapist.

Worksheet 3 'Objective examination of belief', can be used as a template to guide the examination. The questions should be used as a general guide and employed with flexibility. The answers to these questions will lead to ideas for further assignments and behavioural experiments that the client can do with their therapist or as 'homework'. This might include gathering information to support or refute the hypothesis, seeking an independent opinion or reviewing the evidence for its strengths and weaknesses.

Behavioural experiments

Behavioural experiments can be used to objectively examine beliefs in a systematic way. A basic behavioural experiment protocol would be as follows:

1. Identify target belief. What does the person currently believe? (Theory A)
2. Alternative belief. What would be an alternative view? (Theory B)
3. Prediction. What does the person think will happen?
4. Operationalised prediction. How will the prediction be tested?
5. Details of experiment. How is the experiment designed?
6. Results of the experiment. What happened?
7. Conclusion. What was learnt?

An example is presented in Handout 13 'Behavioural experiment: Joe'. Go through this example with the group to illustrate how behavioural experiments can be used to investigate beliefs.

Clients can design their own behavioural experiments on an individual basis with help from their therapist. Copies of Worksheet 4 'Behavioural experiment' can be used as sample worksheets for behavioural experiments.

Level 6: Schema-focused interventions

This level of intervention can be used to explore core beliefs.

Schemata can be conceptualised as the specific cognitive rules that govern information processing and behaviour. They are stable cognitive patterns which screen, differentiate and organise our information. Schemata are formed early in life and are added to and reinforced to build up a stored body of personal knowledge.

Core beliefs can be seen as the most sensitive component of the self-concept, for example if a person views themselves as vulnerable, helpless, inept and so on, this impacts on all aspects of their life. Such underlying core beliefs are generally viewed as components of schemata. Thus schemata are broad, pervasive themes about oneself and one's relationship with others. They are deeply entrenched patterns central to one's sense of self, usually self-perpetuating and difficult to change (Young, 1991).

Schema-focused cognitive therapy was developed in order to help clients with deeply entrenched core beliefs, often those diagnosed as having a personality disorder or other apparently intractable problems. The techniques of schema-focused cognitive therapy have been used to help people understand how they view their world, how childhood influences have impacted on their thinking, and how to adopt new ways of understanding themselves and their behaviour. Identifying core beliefs and schemata can help a person to understand their problems and how dysfunctional beliefs affect their lives. For example, a schema such as vulnerability might lead the person to believe that other people are potential threats, that the future is unpredictable and frightening and that they are helpless and dependent on others.

Working at this level of intervention with people with a diagnosis of schizophrenia can be beneficial if dysfunctional core beliefs are identified. The following exercise based on 'Schema as Self Prejudice' (Padesky, 1993) allows the client to examine their own dysfunctional beliefs and review the evidence for them.

Doubt versus certainty in core beliefs

This exercise can be completed using a common prejudice in order to illustrate the technique. Once this is established, the exercise can be repeated using the person's own identified core belief.

1 Ask the client to identify a belief, which they hold strongly, for example women are bad drivers.

2 Ask them how they would react if they read in the newspaper that new statistics showed more accidents are caused by women drivers than by men.
   – they would be likely to accept this as it confirms their belief
   – they would be likely to have good recollection of the article
   – the belief would be strengthened.

3 Ask how they would react if they read an article showing that men cause more accidents than women.
   – they would be likely to ignore it or to 'rubbish the article'
   – they might recall counter examples
   – they would be more likely to forget the article.

4 Ask how they would react to a neutral article on road safety and gender.
   – they might distort this information to fit their beliefs about female drivers.

5 Ask the person to imagine that their belief was beginning to cause problems. For example, they became dependent on a lift to work from a female colleague during a public transport strike. How might they overcome their belief?
   – they might use the opportunity to gather counter evidence
   – exposure to a good woman driver might help to question the belief.

6 Ask whether this one example will change their belief:
   – it is unlikely as such beliefs are deepseated and need constant vigilance in order to question and change. Any key evidence can trigger a re-emergence of the belief.

This exercise can be repeated with the identified core belief. This provides very helpful information about what maintains the beliefs and how the belief might be changed or modified. It helps the client to distance themselves from the belief and identifies further work that might help to reduce the strength of the core belief. Psychological interventions using schema-focused cognitive therapy requires specialist training in this approach.

Common environmental and mood state precipitants

Environmental	Mood state
Noise level	Happy
Number of people	Sad
Activity level	Upset
Familiar/unfamiliar	Angry
Demanding	Tense
Friends/strangers	Calm
	Confused
	Preoccupied
	Frightened

Hallucination monitoring record

Date	**Environment, eg no of people**	**Mood, eg tense**	**Hallucination present/absent**
am			
pm			
Evening			

Personal questionnaire

Example 1

Name *Peter Ellis*

Week *1 January–*

Delusion/belief *My parents are impostors*

Rating scale *0%–100%*

Rating frequency *Once per month*

1 How certain are you?

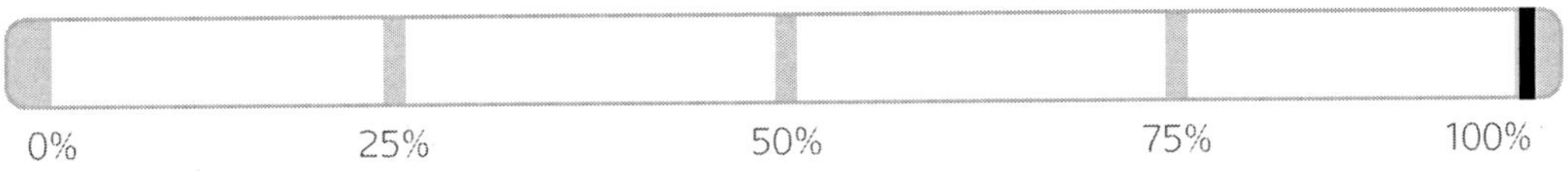

2 How important is this to you?

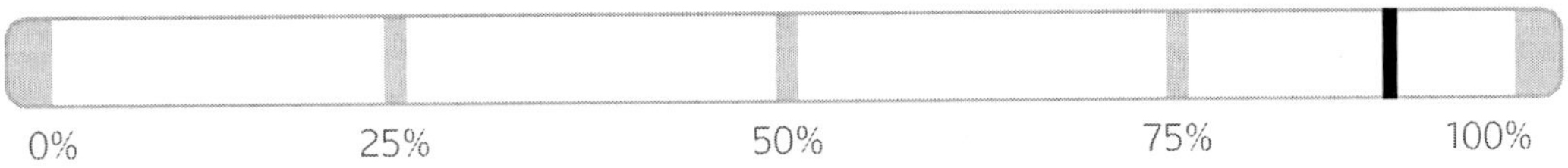

3 How much of the time do you think about this?

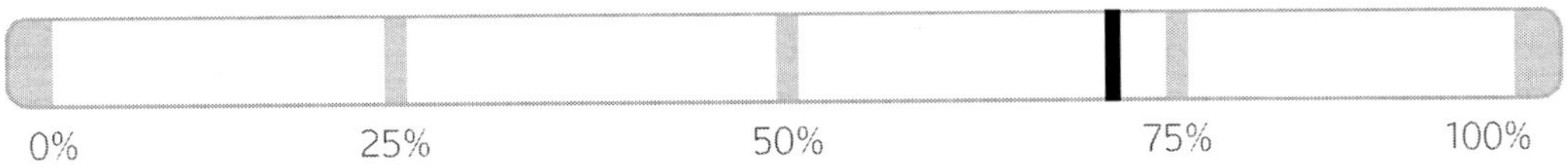

4 How upset does this make you?

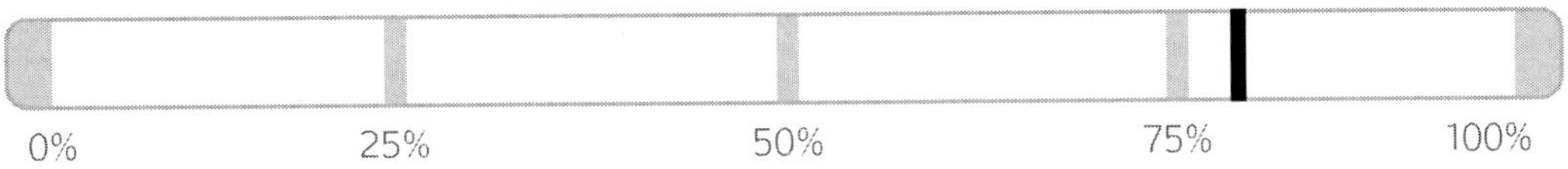

5 How well do you cope with this?

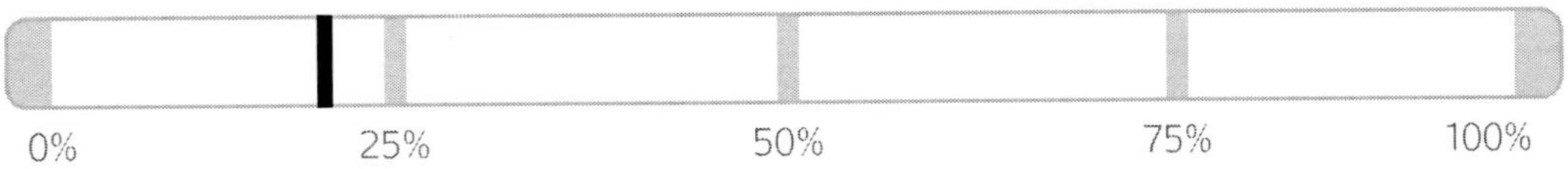

Personal questionnaire

Example 2

Name *Roger Wood*

Week *1 Jan – 7 Jan*

Delusion/belief *People know what I am thinking*

Rating scale *1–5*

Rating frequency *Once per week*

In the past week

- How often have you experienced this?

1 (Not at all) 2 3 (4 circled) 5 (All the time)

- How much have you believed it?

1 (Not at all) 2 3 4 (5 circled) (Completely)

- How much distress has it caused you?

1 (Not at all) 2 3 (4 circled) 5 (Extreme)

- How often have you thought about it?

1 (Not at all) 2 3 (4 circled) 5 (All the time)

Diary sheet for monitoring symptoms

Day	Symptom, eg voice	Situation	Coping response	Effectiveness (1–10)
Monday				
Tuesday				
Wednesday				
Thursday				
Friday				
Saturday				
Sunday				

How we cope with positive symptoms

Take 'prn' medication

Listen to music

Try not to think about it

Go to bed

Watch television

Dance

Relaxation

Think about other things

Talk to someone

Go for a walk

Put headphones on

Argue with the voices

Earplugs

Tell voices to go away

Sing, hum

Categories of coping strategies

Behavioural strategies

- Distraction techniques — 'hum'
  'sing'
- Reducing stimulation — 'go to bed'
- Physical activity — 'dance'
- Direct action — 'ear plugs'
  'headphones'
  'shout'
  'listen to radio/TV'

Cognitive strategies

- Distraction techniques — 'try not to think about it'
- Thought switching — 'think of other things'
- Direct challenge — 'tell voices to go away'
  'argue with voices'

Environmental strategies

- Increase social contact — 'talk to someone'
- Change environment — 'go for a walk'

Physiological strategies

- Medication
- Change mood — 'dance'
- Change arousal — 'relaxation'

More coping strategies for hallucinations

There are many different ways of actively coping with auditory and visual hallucinations. You might have your own techniques, here are some that people have found helpful:

- Challenge the reality; ask yourself if your mind might be 'playing tricks' especially if:
  - you are very tired
  - you are taking drugs
  - you are very upset or confused
- Gain control: challenge the voices, ignore them, tell them to go away
- Set limits: only listen for a short time
- Listen selectively: listen to the positive voices; ignore/challenge the negative voices
- Communicate: talk about your experiences with professionals; get support from family and friends
- Distance yourself from the experiences: write down the experiences, make notes on the physical characteristics, content, etc
- Change your situation: try to refocus, meditate, relax
- Remember your coping strategy enhancement work

Ten ways we get things wrong (page 1 of 2)

1 **Self-serving basis**

We tend to pay more attention to situations which are consistent with our beliefs; this reinforces our beliefs. We prove that we are right, eg someone who believes that women should stay at home to look after their children would be likely to take notice of an article agreeing with this view.

2 **Selective attention**

We ignore or dismiss evidence which contradicts our beliefs, eg someone who believes that mothers should stay at home would find reasons for criticising evidence that children of working mothers did equally well or better at school.

3 **Perceived intentionality**

We misinterpret events based on our assumption that people behaved in a certain way 'on purpose' or deliberately rather than as a function of lack of knowledge, accident or mistake, eg a child who breaks her sister's toy.

4 **Mitigating factors**

Our capacity for making judgements is impaired by a variety of factors, which we seldom take into account. These factors include heightened emotions, tiredness, stress, alcohol, ill health.

5 **Superstition**

We often look for 'hidden meanings' and act on 'intuition' or 'gut feeling', especially if we have limited information or evidence.

Ten ways we get things wrong (page 2 of 2)

6 **Judgement bias**

We rarely act like scientists working out a situation using evidence, likelihoods and probabilities. Rather we are more likely to take account of personalised views, eg one in three marriages end in divorce, but most people marry believing that their marriage will last forever.

7 **Prejudice/stereotyping**

This arises from our need to categorise people and order our world. We all hold common stereotypes to a greater or lesser degree, eg 'men with shaved heads and tattoos are aggressive'.

8 **Isolated incidents**

Even apparently small incidents can have a lasting effect on our judgements, and are selectively reinforced, eg a child who was chased by a dog might develop a fear of dogs. If that child avoids dogs thereafter he or she will never have any positive experiences with dogs to challenge the belief.

9 **Memory errors**

We do not record and review our experiences like a video camera. Our memories are often distorted by subsequent events and can affect the way we view present events, eg a person who believed they were uncared for as a child might fail to recall positive events such as childhood birthday parties.

10 **Thinking errors**

We are subject to a number of common thinking errors which can lead to biases and inaccuracies. These are described in Handout 8 'Common thinking errors'.

Common thinking errors (page 1 of 2)

Our thoughts are not true reflections of reality, they are not 'right' or 'wrong' but are our interpretations of reality.

1 **All-or-nothing thinking**

This is a tendency to think in absolute extremes. In fact very few situations are black and white, although it is often harder for us to see grey. We tend to view situations as 'either/or' rather than 'both', eg 'He is really evil'.

2 **Overgeneralising**

This is the tendency to assume something is always the case because it has happened once, eg making one driving error: 'I am a really bad driver'.

3 **Personalising**

This is the tendency to have an unrealistic sense of responsibility, or exaggerate our role in situations. We might relate everything that happens to ourselves even if it has little or nothing to do with us, eg 'It's my fault no one is enjoying themselves'. Sometimes extreme personalising can lead people to believe they are responsible for completely unrelated events such as disasters, plane crashes, etc.

4 **Fixed rules**

People with excessively high standards and expectations set up rules for themselves and others which are impossible to meet, eg one should always be on time.

Common thinking errors (page 2 of 2)

5 **Catastrophising**

This is the tendency to magnify and exaggerate negative aspects of a situation. Blowing things out of all proportion is a common thinking error. In extreme cases catastrophising can include disastrous thoughts about the whole world.

6 **Ignoring the positives**

People often ignore the positive aspects of situations, concentrate on the negative aspects and even change positives into negatives', eg 'He only said I look nice because he feels sorry for me'.

7 **Predicting the future**

This is the tendency to imagine outcomes to events or situations that have not yet happened. When we predict the future we are extrapolating from limited information and past experiences. We are not looking at reality because it has not yet happened.

8 **Jumping to conclusions**

This is using insufficient evidence or even no evidence at all, eg the reason she did not phone is because she thinks I'm a bad person. This is sometimes called 2 + 2 = 5 thinking.

Examining beliefs vignette: Bill

Bill, a 42-year-old father of four children, heard on the local television news that a consignment of illegal drugs worth over £1 million had been seized at Heathrow airport. The drugs had been flown in from Jamaica.

Later that week his eldest son, Sam, aged 13, went to play at Jamie, his best friend's house. When Sam returned he told his father excitedly that Jamie's father was an airline pilot based at Heathrow airport. Sam talked to his father about Jamie's father a great deal over the following weeks; about the places he flies to, including Jamaica, his sports car, and their new house with a swimming pool.

Sam is an athletic boy who has been selected to represent his school in a county triathlon event. He spends more and more time at Jamie's. One evening he returns home looking very pale and sweaty, and goes straight to bed. Over the following weeks Sam spends a lot of time on his own in his bedroom, and is out at Jamie's house. He starts wearing a long-sleeved football shirt all the time and refuses to wear a short-sleeved T-shirt that his mother bought him. He has become sullen and moody and has developed facial acne.

Bill suddenly has a terrible realisation that Jamie's father is a drug trafficker who is injecting Sam with heroin.

How to improve judgements

1. Ask other people what they think about the situation.
2. What is the evidence? Gather as much as you can.
3. What alternative explanations are there?
4. What contrary evidence are you not considering?
5. What is the effect of thinking this way? How does it make you feel; if it elicits strong emotions check for thinking errors.
6. Are you making any thinking errors, eg jumping to conclusions, personalising, exaggerating the importance of events?
7. Is your belief based on fact or opinion?
8. What are the advantages and disadvantages of thinking this way?

Remember that you might need help to look for alternative explanations and contrary evidence, so talk to someone that you trust.

Case vignette: Jane

Jane is a 34-year-old woman with a 10-year history of contact with psychiatric services. She lives on her own in a flat where she has been for one year. In recent months Jane has become increasingly distressed by her belief that she is under police surveillance, and that she is being videoed via police helicopters and speed cameras. She has mentioned this to several people but no one believes her. She is becoming suspicious of other people and wonders if they are 'in on it' when they do not believe her.

Jane has gathered evidence for her belief, for example she has noted that helicopters sometimes circle overhead and that new speed cameras have been erected on the road that she frequently uses. This has strengthened her conviction that she is right. She has not looked at alternative explanations or the contrary evidence.

Jane has become constantly vigilant and avoids going out if she thinks a helicopter might be out. She has lost her job because of taking days off. She is becoming increasingly anxious and depressed.

Objective examination of belief: Jane (page 1 of 3)

My belief: I am under surveillance; police are videoing me from helicopters and speed cameras.

1 What do other people think?

- People think I am wrong.
- People think I am joking or that I'm mad.
- No one holds this belief or agrees with me.
- When people try to argue with me or say it is not possible, I think perhaps they are involved in the surveillance operation.

2 What is the evidence?

- There are frequently helicopters flying over my flat.
- Sometimes I see the same helicopters when I am out shopping.
- Sometimes the helicopters circle overhead.
- Speed cameras have been fitted on the road I use to walk to the shops.

3 What alternative explanations are there?

- Perhaps the helicopters are doing something else.
- Jane and her therapist decide that Jane should ask a friend to telephone the local RAF base; they told her that they do day and night-time exercise flights.
- Perhaps the speed cameras are used to reduce speeding.
- Jane was asked to contact the local council who provided information on the siting of speed cameras; they were on busy areas such as near schools and shops, and accident 'black spots'.

Objective examination of belief: Jane (page 2 of 3)

4 What is the contrary evidence?

- The helicopters have been flying for several years, but I only moved here last year.
- Sometimes I hear the helicopters in the distance but they don't fly over the flats.
- The speed cameras are often covered up or vandalised; they would be fixed more quickly if they were for surveillance.

5 What is the effect of thinking this way?

- How this makes me feel: upset, angry, scared.
- How this affects me physically: my heart races when I hear helicopters. I become sweaty and hot when I pass speed cameras.
- How this affects my behaviour: I am constantly vigilant. I avoid going out if I have heard a helicopter. I avoid roads with speed cameras.
- How this affects my relationships: people think I am strange. I have disagreements and arguments. I have lost friends. I am suspicious of people.
- How this affects other areas of my life: I cannot go to work. I lost my job.

6 Thinking errors

- I might be jumping to conclusions. There is no direct evidence linking the helicopters or cameras to surveillance.
- I might be personalising. It is true that there are many other people in the vicinity of the helicopter flight path. There are 25 other people in this block of flats.
- The camera is not outside my flat, it is on a busy road.

Objective examination of belief: Jane (page 3 of 3)

7 Am I confusing a fact with an opinion?

- There is no direct link between the helicopters or cameras and me, it is my assumption.
- I monitored helicopter flights; there were four in the last 3-week period, this is not as frequent as I had thought.
- I have no direct evidence or proof that I am under surveillance.

8 Advantages and disadvantages

- I thought it was an advantage to be constantly vigilant, but it just makes me upset and scared.
- There are lots of disadvantages in all the ways it affects me.

Objective examination of belief (page 1 of 3)

My belief

1 What do other people think?
- When you talk about your belief with other people what sort of reaction do you get?
- Does anyone else hold the belief? If so are they agreeing because they are a friend or are they independent?
- If someone does not hold the belief why do you think that is?

2 What is the evidence?
List all the evidence for your belief below:

3 What alternative explanations are there?
You might need to ask other people.

Objective examination of belief (page 2 of 3)

4 What is the contrary evidence?

Remember we tend to be selective in looking at evidence that fits our hypothesis/belief. We need to make an effort to look at what does not fit.

List any contrary evidence below:

5 What is the effect of thinking this way?

- How this makes me feel ...
- How this affects me physically ...
- How this affects my behaviour ...
- How this affects my relationships ...
- How this affects other areas of my life ...

Objective examination of belief (page 3 of 3)

6 Thinking errors

- Am I exaggerating the importance of events?
- Am I jumping to conclusions — this is sometimes described as 2 + 2 = 5 thinking. Can you see any gaps in how you came to your conclusions.
- Am I taking things too personally?

7 Am I confusing a fact with an opinion?

Remember that facts are true and can be demonstrated or proved. Opinions are judgements or personal views.

8 Advantages and disadvantages.

List all the advantages and all the disadvantages of holding this belief below:

Behavioural experiment: Joe (page 1 of 2)

1 Target belief

Joe believes that when he looks into people's eyes he can see himself and this means that he is receiving a message from the devil, therefore he is evil.

(Theory A)

2 Alternative belief

Eyes reflect the images in front of them. If anyone looks closely into someone else's eyes they will see themselves reflected.

(Theory B)

3 Prediction

Joe predicts that he is the only one who can see himself when he looks into people's eyes, so he must be in league with the devil.

4 Operational prediction

If Theory A is correct only Joe will be able to see himself in other people's eyes. If Theory B is correct other people will have the same experience.

5 The experiment

Conduct a survey of five people, such as family, friends. Ask them: if you look very closely into someone's eyes do you see yourself? (They might have to test this out if they had not noticed before.)

Behavioural experiment: Joe (page 2 of 2)

6 Results

Put a tick or a cross for each person's answer to the survey:

Person	Sees self in other's eyes
1	✓
2	✓
3	✓
4	✓
5	✓

7 Conclusion

Theory B was proven; Theory A was not proven.

Behavioural experiment (page 1 of 2)

1 Target belief

What do you currently believe (Theory A)?

2 Alternative belief

What might be an alternative view (Theory B)?

3 Prediction

What do you think would happen?

4 Operational prediction

How will the prediction be tested?

Behavioural experiment (page 2 of 2)

5 The experiment

Detail how the experiment will be set up.

6 Results

What happened?

7 Conclusion

What was learnt?

MODULE 4

Maximising mental health

Overview of Module

- Introduction
- Improving interpersonal effectiveness
- Problem solving
- Problem solving practice
- Interpersonal skills
- Goal planning
- Coping with stress
- Coping with negative symptoms
- Medication

Suggested Session Plans

Problem solving steps	**10 min**
Problem solving example	**30 min**
Problem solving practice exercise	**30 min**
Action step role play	**20 min**
Interpersonal skills practice sessions:	**allow 45 minutes per skill**
Discussion: emotions and cognitions in interpersonal skills	**25 min**
Techniques for improving interpersonal performance	**25 min**
Compilation of social situation practice hierarchy	**40 min**
Goal planning steps	**15 min**
Goal planning example	**15 min**
Personal goal plan	**1 hour**
Identifying stressors exercise	**15 min**
Personal identification of stressors	**20 min**
Stress tracking example	**20 min**
Constructing stress tracker	**20 min**
Anticipating stress example and discussion	**15 min**
Introduction to personal stress awareness	**5 min**
Stress signs and signals	**15 min**
Personal signs and signals of stress	**10 min**
Coping with stress discussion	**15 min**
Strategies for coping with stress	**15 min**
Stress coping records	**15 min**
Review and question and answer session	**15 min**
Introduction to negative symptoms	**15 min**
Personal experiences of the 'big three'	**15 min**
Activity schedules example	**15 min**
Preparation of personal activity schedules	**15 min**
Graded exposure hierarchy intervention	**30 min**
Supplementary individual sessions required	
Non-adherence to prescribed medication, guided learning	**30 min**
Non-adherence to antipsychotic medication, guided discussion	**30 min**
Exploring personal reasons for non-adherence	**30 min**
Experiences of prescribed medication	**30 min**
Exploration to improve adherence – individual	**1 hour**
Medication review – individual	**1 hour**

Introduction

This module focuses on enhancing those factors which might 'protect' against the development of future episodes of illness or reduce the impact of such episodes as well as improving quality of life. The vulnerability stress model suggests that both environmental factors such as life events and emotional atmosphere, and personal factors such as coping ability, self-efficacy and interpersonal abilities are important in maintaining good mental health. In addition to their protective role factors such as interpersonal skills, communication and self-management skills can increase the overall level of social, occupational and personal functioning. The module covers four areas: improving interpersonal effectiveness, coping with stress, coping with negative symptoms and medication.

Improving interpersonal effectiveness

The majority of our day-to-day problems, 'hassles' and difficulties arise from our dealings with other people. There is a need to communicate with people in all aspects of our lives: at work, with family and friends, and in activities of daily living such as shopping, recreation and healthcare. Having an ability to deal effectively with other people makes life easier!

Classical family intervention work has focused on areas of social functioning and communication, in particular addressing high 'expressed emotion' in relatives. Expressed emotion is a good short-term predictor of relapse in people with a diagnosis of schizophrenia who are living at home. Family interventions, while addressing the relationship between relative/carer and the person with schizophrenia tend to focus on improving the relative or carer's ability to 'cope with' the patient and difficulties associated with caring. Typical interventions include focused problem solving, education, coping with problem behaviours and symptoms. While this approach is often very helpful, it tends not to fully examine the issues from the perspective of the person with the diagnosis of schizophrenia. The current programme emphasises the client's perspective in working collaboratively with key people in their lives and enhancing their skills in order to improve interpersonal effectiveness.

It is a common assumption that due to lack of 'insight' people with a diagnosis of schizophrenia not only fail to recognise that they are 'ill' but also fail to identify other problems in their lives, such as interpersonal difficulties. Frequently, the person's problems are identified by mental health professionals, for example the need for social skills training, or it is assumed that they will have deficits, for example in communication. However, people with a diagnosis of schizophrenia have been found to have good insight into the severity of their interpersonal problems in general. It has also been found that insight into interpersonal problems is not associated with insight into 'illness' (Startup, 1998).

Interpersonal functioning problems might be one of the first 'prodromal signs' which are noticed by the person themself as well as by other people. Avoidance of social contact, reduction in communication and decline in other interpersonal abilities can signal the onset of an acute phase, and also remain as ongoing problems. DSM-IV diagnostic criteria include impairments in social functioning in the description of schizophrenia.

Improving interpersonal effectiveness can be achieved by three main strategies: problem solving, interpersonal skills and goal planning.

Problem solving

Introduce this topic to the group by explaining that problems are often perpetuated by inaction, avoidance or unhelpful strategies such as arguing or blaming others. Taking a positive view of problems as difficulties which can be solved, is empowering and can also alleviate stress and help us to feel more in control of our lives. The best way to solve a problem is to follow a basic strategy which assists in thinking rationally and thoroughly about the problem. This strategy helps to examine options and the consequences of different solutions before a course of action is planned and carried out.

On a flipchart draw seven columns in ascending steps. As you talk through the problem solving strategy write the name of each step in the appropriate column. Keep the description simple and clear. Further discussion and practice of each step will follow.

- Step 1: define the problem
- Step 2: stop and think
- Step 3: gather information
- Step 4: generate alternatives
- Step 5: think about the consequences

- Step 6: planning
- Step 7: action

Ensure that the group understands the steps and invite questions and comments. Provide clients with Handout 1, 'The problem solving strategy', before going through the strategy step by step using the following example.

Phil, a young man with a diagnosis of schizophrenia has recently moved into shared accommodation with three other residents. One of them, Tom, plays loud music and it is disturbing Phil.

Step 1

Define the problem. Ask the group: What is Phil's problem? Make sure that this is defined in terms of where he is now and where he wants to be. More than one possible definition might be suggested, if so discuss the differences between them and decide which problem you are going to work on. In defining the problem ensure that you do not jump to solutions, for example Phil does not like being in a flat, he wants to move out. In this example the most straightforward definition of the problem is: Phil is being disturbed by loud music (where he is now), Phil does not want to be disturbed by loud music (where he wants to be).

Step 2

Stop and think. Ask the group why Phil needs to stop and think, and what he needs to think about. He needs to stop and think in order to avoid acting impulsively and leaping to a solution. This also helps him to avoid acting on 'hot' emotions such as anger. He needs to think about what information he might need, what other people think and what alternatives he might have.

Step 3

Seek information. Ask the group who would be a good source of information and what Phil should find out. Phil should ask the other residents what they think about Tom playing loud music. He needs to find out how long it has been going on for, if anyone else finds this a problem, and whether anyone has talked to him about it. He could also ask his social worker about what he could do.

Step 4

Generate alternatives. Ask the group what Phil's options are. Brainstorm all the alternatives, no ideas are criticised at this stage, just try to generate as many ideas as possible. Possible alternatives would include: ask Tom to turn his music down; move out; break his CD player; Phil could play his music louder; buy earplugs; enlist the help of other residents to tell Tom to turn his music down.

Step 5

Think about the consequences. What are the costs and benefits of these options? Ask the group to select two alternatives and do a cost–benefit analysis on each. These are illustrated in Figure 4. Having worked through

Option 1: Ask Tom to turn his music down

	Benefit	Cost
Short-term	It might work and he will turn music down Feel good that have said something/been assertive	It might not work and he could get annoyed It is hard to ask as do not know him well
Long-term	Improve communication Feel pleased that can be assertive If this works — no more loud music	Loss of potential friendship

Option 2: Play music louder

	Benefit	Cost
Short-term	Feel have 'got even'	Tom could turn his music louder Might cause worse conflict Annoy other residents
Long-term	None	Ongoing feud Might be asked to leave Ongoing bad feeling Does not solve problem

Figure 4 Cost–benefit analysis example

both cost–benefit analyses ask the group which is the preferred option. If neither is satisfactory, they can choose another option or go back and gather more information.

Step 6

Planning. Ask the group what Phil should consider in planning. He needs to consider when to ask Tom (if this is the preferred option!). He needs to find a quiet time when Tom is not busy. He needs to plan what to say; he could practise this with a friend.

Step 7

Action. Ask the group what Phil has to do. He has to carry out the plan and see if it works. Ask the group to give feedback and comments about the strategy and how it might be used in practice.

Problem solving practice

Group members should be given the opportunity to practise the seven-step approach using their own problems. This can be carried out in pairs with assistance from facilitators as required. The primary aim is to practise the strategy and to become familiar with the process. Clients should therefore be encouraged to choose a current or recent problem that they could share with the group, for example being asked to lend money to a friend. Discourage complex or ongoing problems for analysis at this stage, such as problematic relationships. Allow approximately 30 minutes for this exercise. Each pair should decide on the problem they will work on. Provide flipchart paper for clients to outline each step and assist in their feedback to the group. This exercise can then be repeated to enable each individual to work through their own problem in pairs.

Step 7, the action step, should then be practised. This is carried out as a whole group exercise. Ask for a volunteer to briefly summarise their chosen problem and solution, and how they plan to carry out the solution. They should then choose a fellow role player and go through the action step in role play. Following the role play, which is likely to take two to three minutes, ask the person how successful they think they were and what they might try to do differently. Invite feedback from the group. Each person should take a turn to practise their action step in front of the group.

Encourage clients to use this strategy with other problems which might arise over the following weeks, and invite them to discuss this in individual sessions with their therapist.

Interpersonal skills

Finding a solution to a problem is not enough. In order to carry out the solution effectively, interpersonal skills are needed. It might have become apparent during the problem-solving role plays that skills such as assertiveness, perspective taking and managing emotions are important.

The best way to learn interpersonal skills is to understand the rules of such skills, watch them in action and then practise them. Interpersonal skills sessions should follow this process:

1. Introduce the skill and outline the skill steps involved.
2. Facilitators role play a scenario in front of the group to illustrate the use of the skill steps.
3. Ask the group for personal examples of where they might use this skill.
4. Provide the opportunity for practising the skill by clients role playing their examples in pairs, with facilitator feedback.

Schedule a number of interpersonal skills practice sessions. The particular skills chosen will, of course, depend on the needs of the client group.

Interpersonal skills sessions should be tailored to the needs of the individual group members. The main objectives are to enhance existing skills and to promote self-confidence in dealing with social situations. It is therefore important to create a safe and positive atmosphere where people are rewarded by praise and encouragement, and are given plenty of opportunity to refine and practise their skills. Clients' own examples of situations provide the best scenarios for role play and practice. Skill steps and example scenarios for facilitator demonstrations are provided in Box 4.

BOX 4 Skill steps for interpersonal effectiveness
(based on work of Arnold P Goldstein, *The Prepare Curriculum*, 1999)

Asking for help

1 What is the problem that you need help with?
2 Decide if you need help to solve the problem
3 Choose who might be able to help
4 Tell the person about your problem and ask them for help

Example: Day care nursery is closing down, need help to solve childcare problem. Choose a person with similar experience and ask if they have any advice.

Giving instructions

1 Decide what needs to be done
2 Think about the people who could do it and choose someone
3 Explain how to do it
4 Ask the person if they understand what to do
5 Repeat the instructions if you need to

Example: Person is going away for a weekend and needs someone to look after their pet. Instructions will include feeding, exercise and routine.

Apologising

1 Decide if it would be best to apologise for something you did
2 Think of different ways you could apologise; say something, do something, write something
3 Choose the best time and place
4 Make your apology which might include a way of making up for what happened

Example: Apologise to a friend for betraying a confidence.

Listening

1 Pay attention to the person talking
2 Think about what the person is saying
3 Do not interrupt; wait your turn to speak
4 Say what you want to say

Example: Listen to flatmate telling you why they did not do the washing up last night.

BOX 4 *continued*

Convincing others

1 Decide specifically what you want someone to do
2 Choose the right person to ask and decide why they would want to do what you are asking
3 State what you want them to do and why
4 Ask for their reaction
5 Present additional reasons

Example: Convince your doctor that you are ready to have home leave from hospital.

Assertiveness

1 Think about what you want to say
2 Be clear and concise
3 Tell the person how you feel
4 Tell the person what you would like to be different
5 Try to use 'I' rather than 'you', for example 'I feel upset' not 'you make me upset'

Example: Tell your boss that you have too much to do and would like some help.

Responding to failure

1 Decide if you have failed at something
2 Think about why you failed
3 Think about what you could do differently
4 Decide if you want to try again
5 Try again using your new idea

Example: Failing a driving test.

Negotiation

1 Decide if you and the other person are having a difference of opinion
2 Tell the person what you think about the problem
3 Ask the person what they think about the problem
4 Listen openly to their answer
5 Think about why they might feel this way
6 Suggest a compromise

Example: Your flatmate thinks that you are not doing your fair share of household chores.

BOX 4 *continued*

Responding to persuasion

1 Listen to the person's ideas on a topic
2 Decide what you think about a topic
3 Compare what the other person has said to what you think
4 Decide which idea you prefer and tell the person your decision

Example: You are being persuaded to sell your music centre.

Emotions and cognitions in interpersonal skills

Having practised a range of interpersonal skills and learnt the skill steps to be followed, skills can be further refined by paying attention to the sources of intrapersonal difficulties, which can inhibit good social skills. These are essentially the person's own feelings and thoughts.

Explain to the group that often the reasons for poor performance in social situations are what we are feeling, for example embarrassment, anxiety, tension, anger and what we are thinking, for example 'I look foolish', 'They think I'm stupid', 'He does not like me'. The key to overcoming these barriers to effective interpersonal skills is preparation: by anticipating likely thoughts and feelings that particular situations might evoke, we can develop coping strategies to deal with them in advance. The more we practise in imagination, the easier real-life situations become.

Ask the group to give examples of situations they find particularly difficult. These might include speaking in public, conflict or disagreement, meeting new people, social gatherings, talking to authority figures. Ask the group to imagine that they are in a situation that they find difficult and ask why they find these situations difficult. Ask them to imagine how they will feel and what they will think. This is likely to elicit a series of self-doubts or fears, which could be listed on a flipchart, placing thoughts in one column and feelings in another. Common examples are likely to include: 'I will go red', 'I won't know what to say', 'I will stutter', 'They will think I'm strange', 'I will get anxious'. Point out that this illustrates how easy it is to imagine future scenarios and to see oneself not coping. Such negative anticipation reinforces poor performance and increases the likelihood of this happening. In order to counteract this problem there are a number of strategies to practise in imagination, in role play and in real-life situations. The strategies include: positive self-statements, thought switching, body language, acting 'as if', covert relaxation and breathing and calming techniques. Provide clients with Handout 2, 'Improving interpersonal performance', and talk through each strategy.

In order to practise these strategies, help clients to construct a short hierarchy of difficult situations that they would like to work on. Starting with the least difficult, talk through what they are likely to say to themselves to make the situation worse, and compile a series of positive self-statements to counteract this. Similarly, ask them to identify negative emotions which might be evoked and plan how they will cope with these using any of the above strategies. Once a series of coping strategies have been identified the person should practise them, first in imagination and second by role playing the situation. Real-life 'behavioural experiments' can then be set up to enable the person to practise their skills. Ensure that the tasks that are set are achievable and are at an appropriate level in the hierarchy before progressing on to more difficult situations.

Goal planning

Goal planning is a commonly used strategy in family interventions. This is a strategy which helps to find solutions to situations that are causing distress or disagreement, or are simply holding back the person from achieving success. It is particularly useful in situations which have reached an apparent impasse, or which are destructive, self-defeating or perpetuated by avoidance.

Explain the principles of goal planning to the group. There are four basic steps.

Step 1

Establish the goals. This involves drawing up a short list of what the person would like to achieve. These should be short-term, ie one to three months, or medium-term, six to twelve months. Having drawn up the list, an order of priority should be established. The person should address one goal at a time, selecting the easiest or the most urgent with which to start. It is likely that the goal will involve another person such as the person's partner, relative or carer, in which case the collaborative involvement of the person might be sought in order to help in setting the goal.

Step 2

Operationalise the goal. Having selected a goal to work on it should be made as specific as possible. If it is too generalised it will be difficult to attain. For example a goal of 'working harder' would be difficult to define and should be made more specific, for example spend two hours per day on computer course. The person should then draw up a brief action plan of how the goal will be achieved. This may contain one or two stages of the plan or might involve a more detailed breakdown of the steps to be followed.

It is also helpful to be able to measure the achievement of the goal, therefore a way of measuring success should be built into the establishment of the goal. For example, keep a diary or checklist of whether the action plan has been followed. Lastly, in this step, ensure that the goal set is given a specific timeframe, that is, set a time by which realistically some success might be achieved. The goal can then be reviewed at this point, for example one week, one month or three months, as appropriate.

Step 3

Carry out the plan. Having clarified a specific goal, drawn up a brief action plan, determined that the goal is attainable and measurable and when it will be reviewed, the next step is to carry out the plan.

Step 4

Evaluate success. At the allotted review time the goal should be reviewed by examining how it was measured and carried out and how successful it was. If the goal was fully achieved this should be acknowledged. If it was not fully achieved, the reasons for this should be reviewed: perhaps it was unrealistic and needs to be broken down into smaller more attainable steps. If no progress was made perhaps other issues need to be addressed, such as motivation and whether the goal is important to the person.

Illustrate this process by talking through the example provided in Handout 3, 'Planning goals'.

Clients should be given the opportunity to examine their own goals and to draw up a plan with assistance from the facilitators. Individual plans can be documented using Worksheet 1 'Personal goal plan'. Ensure that the plans are reviewed within the established timeframe and give praise, encouragement and assistance as appropriate. Goal planning is an ongoing process and new goals can be set and planned as current goals are achieved.

Typical areas for goal planning and other solution-focused interventions, include the following:

1. Family – areas of disagreement, irritations, frustrations
2. Housing – accommodation problems, living with others
3. Finances – debt, loans, benefit system, earning money
4. Recreation/social – activities, entertainment, relaxation, social occasions
5. Employment – education, finding a job, skills, dealing with colleagues
6. Interpersonal problems – social role, relationship with carers/professionals, social functioning
7. Daily living – transport, shopping, cooking

Coping with stress

The vulnerability stress model predicts that increases in stress in a vulnerable person will also increase their risk of relapse. It is proposed that acute episodes are triggered by challenging events – primarily environmental stressors. If the person is vulnerable due to genetic or other predispositions, a lower level of stress is sufficient to trigger relapse. However, people can adapt to future potential stressors and learn to reduce their sensitivity to stress.

Identifying stressors

When a person is coping with mental health problems it can be difficult to identify further sources of stress. The effects of external stressors are often amplified by the person's reduced ability to deal with social situations effectively and perhaps by a reduced ability to seek effective help and support.

Explain to the group that the first step in coping effectively with stress is to accurately identify the sources of the stress. Lead a discussion on where stress comes from and ask the group to give general and personal examples. The responses should be listed on a flipchart. It is likely that the sources identified will fall into three main categories: relationships with people; daily living problems; and life events. Point these out to the group. Talk through the information provided in Handout 4 'Identification of stressors', before distributing it to clients.

Note that in addition to the three main sources of external stress, it is also important to identify internal stressors. These are the personal thinking styles, attitudes and beliefs which puts a person 'under pressure' from themself. Examples of this might include perfectionist thinking such as 'I must always do things well', or excessive concerns about the evaluations of other people, for example 'If I get things wrong I will look like a fool'. It is likely that some of these maladaptive thinking patterns have been identified in the interpersonal skills section.

Clients should be assisted in completing Worksheet 2 'Personal identification of stressors', which will help them to clarify current stressors. The worksheet covers each of the main areas of stress in detail, and is likely to require individual guidance from facilitators.

Monitoring stress

Explain to the group that any change we experience can be stressful. Positive as well as negative changes require us to adapt to our new situation. Because of this stress levels fluctuate and it is important to be aware of the increases and decreases in stress, and the effects it has on us. If we are able to monitor our stress levels this can help to ensure that we respond with effective coping strategies.

Stress monitoring includes two main strategies: first, monitoring changes in the sources of the stress, and second, monitoring the effects of stress on the person.

Having successfully identified current sources of stress, clients should be encouraged to keep a simple diary record of changes in these sources. It is likely that two or three primary sources of stress are operating at any one time and tracking these can help to signal when action is required to reduce the effects of stress. An example of stress tracking is shown in Handout 5 'Stress tracking'. Distribute this handout to the group and explain how stress tracking works. The most appropriate monitoring frequency is determined by the type of stressor identified. Stressors that are more consistent, such as concerns about finances, can be sampled less frequently, whereas those that are most changeable, such as arguments with mother, can be sampled more frequently. Stress tracking enables identification of possible patterns and helps to increase the predictability of such stressors; if arguments with mother seem to occur during one-to-one meetings, but not during family meetings, this will help to identify possible action solutions. Similarly, if stress is consistent, for example worrying about finances, this will highlight the need to try to solve such a problem as a priority. Using this example, also point out that while some stress is sudden and unexpected, most stress can be predicted. In the example, it would be possible to predict that the noisy neighbour causes most stress at the end of the week. Perhaps he works between Monday and Thursday, or has celebrations after being paid on a Thursday. Anticipating stress can help clients to prepare for it and take action to reduce its effects. Remind the group of the problem solving strategy which could be used in such situations.

Clients should be assisted to construct their own stress tracking monitoring as appropriate.

In order to assist in anticipating stressors, ask the group to list any stressors they might be able to anticipate occurring in the next three months. This may include items such as those listed in Box 5.

BOX 5 Anticipating stressors, example

Moving ward
Friend going on holiday
Starting work project
Anniversary of mother's death
Sister going into hospital
Christmas
Change in medication
New psychiatrist
Family meeting

The second strategy for monitoring stress involves improving personal stress awareness by noting changes in physical, psychological and behavioural responses. Explain to the group that good awareness of our personal responses to stress can serve as early warning signs that we are under stress and alert us to the need to take action to reduce these effects. Provide clients with Handout 6 'Stress signs and signals'. Talk through each sign and ask clients to note any signals which they recognise as particularly applying to themselves, and to record this on Worksheet 3 'My personal signs and signals of stress'.

Coping strategies

Identifying stressors, monitoring and predicting stress can be helpful in themselves both in reducing the impact of such stress and in highlighting specific coping strategies. Facilitate a group discussion of how people have coped with stress.

Group discussion of personal coping styles and strategies can be very valuable in highlighting successful coping strategies and improving self-efficacy. Drawing on previous similar experiences and illustrating successful coping identifies a range of helpful strategies. All coping strategies suggested should be listed on a flipchart. Unhelpful or potentially damaging strategies such as use of alcohol or illegal drugs, should be discussed in terms of their short term and long term positive and negative consequences. Use this to illustrate that short-term gains are always heavily outweighed by long-term losses. Common personal coping strategies are listed in Box 6.

BOX 6 Coping strategies for stress, example

Talk to a friend
Sleep
Take medication
Talk to psychologist
Ask for help
Relaxation
Listen to music
Go for a walk
Try to solve the problem
Challenge negative thoughts

Present a series of strategies for coping with stress. These are described in Handout 7 'Strategies for coping with stress', which should be distributed after discussion.

Active coping can reduce the impact of stress quite dramatically. In order to maintain coping and increase the likelihood of clients using such strategies it is useful to help construct coping records. These should be simple and easy to fill in, and should be reviewed regularly to illustrate coping success and provide opportunity for positive feedback. An example is provided in Handout 8 'Coping with stress'. This should be talked through with clients before providing the accompanying Worksheet 4 'Coping with stress'. To complete the section on stress, summarise the main learning points and conduct a question and answer session.

Coping with negative symptoms

Reintroduce the idea of negative symptoms and their identification. Explain to the group that negative symptoms of schizophrenia are usually defined by loss or decline in one or more of the following areas: cognitive, social, educational, occupational and personal functioning. Common negative symptoms are listed in Box 7.

BOX 7 Common negative symptoms

Reduced ability to feel and express emotions
Decline in concentration
Reduced speed of information processing
Speech impairments, eg word finding difficulties, impoverished speech
Loss of energy
Lethargy
Loss of enjoyment in activities
Reduced motivation
Loss of initiative
Decline in self-care
Loss of sociability
Loss of enthusiasm

The types of difficulty manifested in the 'negative syndrome' of schizophrenia are similar to those associated with depression, with the side effects of psychotropic medication and with the consequences of experiencing positive symptoms. Detailed assessment and understanding of the presenting difficulties will clarify the nature and extent of symptoms such as social withdrawal, inactivity and loss of motivation. This will help to establish the causes, course, antecedents and consequences of such problems. See Part II and Module 1 for further details. Individual assessment and exploration can clarify whether difficulties are part of a pattern associated with depressed mood or linked with medication side effects, or are as a response to the positive symptoms of schizophrenia. Timeline analysis, mood charts, and so on can be used for this purpose. Interventions for these difficulties encountered by people with a diagnosis of schizophrenia are drawn from cognitive behaviour therapy for people with depression as the presenting problems are very similar, even if the aetiology is different.

Dealing with inactivity, loss of motivation and social withdrawal

Ask the group to provide examples both past and present of their experiences of the type of difficulties described as negative symptoms. These are likely to fall into three general areas: inactivity, loss of motivation and social withdrawal. These are the most commonly cited problems and can be described as 'the big three'.

The consequences of negative symptoms, both for the individual and for those around them, should then be elicited by prompt questions such as: 'How does sitting alone in your room (or other example/difficulty) make you feel?', 'How do other people react when you ...?', 'What have you given up that you used to enjoy?', 'How would things change if you no longer ...?'.

The consequences of such problems often include a reduction in self-esteem, feelings of hopelessness, guilt and feeling overwhelmed. Such problems also frequently evoke negative responses from others who might wrongly interpret the person's behaviour as laziness and therefore react with frustration and criticism.

Explain that it is easy to become trapped in a negative spiral of feeling unable to cope, reduced activity level, feeling tired and hopeless and lacking energy. This physiological change is often accompanied by self-defeating thoughts such as 'I can't do the things I used to', 'I can't be bothered to do things' and 'Everything is such an effort'. Explain that doing less reduces the chances of enjoyment and engagement in activities, and therefore the opportunity for positive reinforcement. Inactivity and loss of motivation can be tackled practically by behaviour change using activity schedules and rewards. It can also be tackled psychologically by thought change such as self-challenging and coping self-statements.

Ask the group for examples to illustrate the point that the more you do, the more you feel like doing. For example, feeling energised after exercise, feeling satisfied after completing a chore. Conversely, ask for examples of doing very little and the subsequent effect, for example staying in bed all day, and feeling more tired and unmotivated.

Activity schedules

Activity schedules are particularly useful for increasing motivation and reducing inactivity. They are records of exact behaviours over specified periods of time, which can be used as a basis for adding to and improving the daily activity. There are six steps in using activity schedules:

1 Keep a daily record of activity for each hour for at least one week.
2 Review the activity schedule for any patterns or points of interest.
3 Explore the consequences of inactivity for yourself and others.
4 Cognitive challenge.
5 Work out a simple action plan to increase activity.
6 Complete another activity schedule for the following week using mastery and pleasure ratings and scheduling in new goal activities.

The use of activity schedules can be illustrated using Handout 9 'Activity schedule: John'. Go through this handout in detail, explaining the six steps and clarifying any points raised.

Mastery ratings are the sense of achievement gained from the activity, and are rated on a ten-point scale: 1 = No sense of achievement, 10 = Great sense of achievement.

Pleasure ratings are the sense of pleasure gained from the activity rated on a 10-point scale; 1 = No sense of pleasure, 10 = Great sense of pleasure.

It is important to ensure that the goal activities are incremental and achievable. Changes should be introduced gradually and new activities introduced at regular intervals. The mastery and pleasure ratings reinforce the idea that the chosen activities do lead to an increased sense of achievement and pleasure. If they do not, change them! There are a wide range of possible activities to consider: for example activities that enhance social, creative, recreational, educational and occupational achievements. Review the activity schedule weekly to reinforce positive changes, 'troubleshoot' any difficulties and discuss alternatives. To assist in choosing pleasurable activities, a list of common activities is provided in Handout 10 'Pleasurable activities'. Blank activity schedules are provided in Worksheet 5 'Activity schedule'.

Social withdrawal

As well as being helpful in increasing motivation and activity levels, the activity schedule process can be used to reduce social withdrawal by scheduling in activities which require social interaction.

Social withdrawal can also be addressed using graded exposure. That is, drawing up a hierarchy of goals, each incrementally more challenging for the person. The hierarchy might include gradually increasing the time spent in social interactions, or increasing the variety of social contacts or the range of social activities. Explain to the group how graded exposure can be used to gradually increase activities based on the individual's own goals. The idea of the hierarchy is to gradually increase the person's ability by incrementally increasing the level of difficulty. Success at one level should be achieved and consolidated before the next level is attempted. An example hierarchy is shown in Box 8. This can be presented to the group by adding each additional level on a flipchart.

BOX 8 Graded exposure hierarchy

Talk to friend (Lyn)

↓

Telephone sister (Mary)

↓

Visit Mary for one hour

↓

Meet Lyn for coffee at home

↓

Meet Lyn for coffee in café

↓

Meet Mary for a meal at home

↓

Meet Mary for a meal in restaurant

↓

Go to Mary's for a day out

↓

Evening out with Lyn

↓

Clients should be helped to construct their own graded hierarchy to work towards achieving a particular social interaction goal.

Medication

If people who have a diagnosis of schizophrenia take antipsychotic medication it reduces their risk of experiencing a further acute episode or relapse in the next year by 60 to 70 per cent (Johnson, 1993). 'Maintenance' medication is commonly prescribed to help prevent people experiencing a re-emergence of their symptoms. A review of research studies of people continuing to take antipsychotic medication versus those not taking it found that over an average of 10 months 16 per cent of patients on medication relapsed, whereas 53 per cent of those not taking medication relapsed (Gilbert et al, 1995). However, even though doctors might explain the likely beneficial effects of antipsychotic medication, and those prescribed it are aware of the reasons to take it, about one-third of people are non-compliant with prophylactic medication for schizophrenia.

This section focuses on the following:

- Understanding individuals' personal experiences of taking medication and not taking medication.
- Discussing antipsychotic medication to improve knowledge and understanding of its likely effects and side effects.
- Interventions to improve the therapeutic alliance between prescriber and prescribee to enhance medication adherence.

Psychiatric patients can be given medication against their will. Many might have experienced involuntary medication while detained under a section of the Mental Health Act. It is not surprising therefore that people with a diagnosis of schizophrenia often feel concerned about being open and honest about their real use of prescribed medication. It is therefore important to create the right conditions to enable people to disclose non-adherence: reducing or stopping medication against the prescriber's advice. The foundations for openness will have been established by building and maintaining a trusting therapeutic relationship and collaborative alliance. In addition, openness can be actively promoted by putting non-adherence in context and exploring the reasons for it.

Understanding non-adherence with prescribed medication

Present the following to the group. It is assumed for all patients, not just those with mental health needs, that taking prescribed medication is in the patient's best interest, and not taking it is detrimental to them. Therefore it is assumed, that people will generally learn to comply with medication because they get better when they do and get worse if they do not. However, these are only two possible outcomes. Draw up the table illustrated in Figure 5 on a flipchart. Write in the outcome: (i), Patient takes medication gets better, and (iv), Patient does not take medication and gets worse. Explain that there are two other possible outcomes. The first is that the medication does not treat the problem adequately, so symptoms might remain or the side effects might make people feel ill. Add this outcome to the chart: (ii), Patient takes medication and does not get better, inadequate or ineffective therapy. Another possible outcome is that the person does not comply with the prescribed medication, stops taking it or reduces it and they get better. Add this to the chart: (iii), Patient does not take medication and gets better. This might occur because of inaccurate diagnosis or overprescription. People's experiences of outcomes (ii) and (iii) on the chart can influence their future likelihood of adhering to prescribed medication.

		Treatment goal	
		Achieved	**Not achieved**
Adherence	High	(i) Patient takes medication and gets better	(ii) Patient takes medication and does not get better, inadequate or ineffective therapy
	Low	(iii) Patient does not take medication and gets better	(iv) Patient does not take medication and gets worse

Figure 5 Adherence and outcomes

Ask the group for examples of their experiences with prescribed medications such as antibiotics. Facilitators could also give their own experiences. A common pattern is that people are prescribed a course of treatment, for example 10 days of antibiotics for an ear infection. Initially adherence is high, however, often the symptoms remit after three to four days and people do not finish the course of medication. Sometimes premature cessation can result in symptoms recurring. Typical adherence with medication for general illnesses is approximately one-third full adherence, one-third partial adherence and one-third non-adherence (Sackett and Haynes, 1976). Point out that people are more likely to comply if they actively present themselves for treatment of a complaint than if, for example they are screened and told to follow up for treatment, such as for high blood pressure or cholesterol level. Those illnesses which require people to take medication over a long period of time or chronic illnesses seem to have similar non-adherence rates to each other. Facilitators should list these illnesses on a flipchart with the percentage rates of non-adherence to prescribed medication next to them, as shown in Box 9.

BOX 9 Non-adherence rates for chronic illnesses

Tuberculosis, 37%
Leprosy, 32%
Diabetes, 42%
Heart failure, 42%
Epilepsy, 37%
Arthritis, 32%

Source: Wright (1993).

Ask the group what percentage of non-adherence to prescribed medication they would estimate for schizophrenia. Reveal that the figure is 33%. This should be discussed in terms of its similarity to other long term problems, which suggests that adherence is not related to 'insight', mental health, and so on, but perhaps it is due to other factors common to chronic illnesses in general.

Having set non-adherence in context, the group should be asked to suggest reasons for non-adherence to prescribed medication in general. These reasons can be listed on a flipchart. Typical responses are listed in Box 10.

BOX 10 Reasons for non-adherence to prescribed medication

Symptoms do not go away
Side effects of medication
Forgetting
Symptoms do go away
Prescription costs
Don't trust the doctor

Facilitate a group discussion concerning additional reasons why people do not adhere to antipsychotic medication, drawing out any personal issues and experiences. The following points should be covered:

- Subjective experience of the drug
  A large study (Hogan et al, 1983) examining the factors which might help to discriminate between adherers and non-adherers found that the person's subjective experience of the drug was the most important factor in predicting adherence. Subjective experience can be positive, for example 'feel more normal', 'thoughts clearer', 'feel more relaxed', and can be negative, for example 'feel like a zombie', 'feel tired and sluggish', 'things more difficult to do'. Therefore, how a person feels on medication, independent of side effects, plays a significant part in whether they will continue to take it. Interestingly, positive subjective experience attributed to neuroleptic medication was the most significant predictor of adherence, with this factor accounting for 59.8 per cent of the total variance. Negative subjective experience accounted for 11.7 per cent and five other factors contributed the remaining variance.
- Health beliefs
  Not surprisingly, disagreement over diagnosis is a factor in non-adherence. People are less likely to comply with medication when they do not believe that they are ill (Marder et al, 1983). Some studies have

found that denial and illness severity are related to non-adherence, although other studies have not found this relationship.

- Attitude to medication
  Beliefs about health, such as 'you take medication when you are ill, not when you are well', do have significant impact on medication non-adherence, particularly in people with illnesses which can remit. Examining this belief in relation to schizophrenia versus other medical problems could be beneficial in increasing adherence. Presenting evidence for the 'maintenance' role of antipsychotic medication is also helpful, that is, continuing to take medication can prevent a relapse and it is therefore important to continue medication even if one feels 'better'.
- Relationship with prescriber
  Interestingly it has been found that adherence to antipsychotic medication is also associated with the therapist liking the patient and believing in the medication (Barofsky and Connelly, 1983). Unresponsiveness to a patient's concerns about side effects might also be related to non-adherence in people with a diagnosis of schizophrenia (Babiker, 1986). Feelings such as being pressured to take medication versus taking it of one's own free will are also likely to influence adherence.
- Beliefs of family/friends
  Higher adherence rates are found in people who are married, have a stable family and are accepted and supported by their family. Adherence is greater if the person is living with a supportive friend or family member who is able to 'supervise' the taking of medication (McEvoy et al, 1989b).
- Medication side effects
  Side effects can include extrapyramidal side effects, sedation, lethargy, dysphoria, sexual dysfunction and weight gain. Occasionally people attribute difficulties such as loss of motivation or dysphoria, erroneously to medication side effects. In such cases adherence can be presented as a behavioural experiment to investigate whether such symptoms improve, stay the same or worsen in response to medication.

Following this discussion Handout 11 'Reasons for non-adherence', should be distributed.

Clients can be assisted to work individually or in pairs in order to examine personal reasons, if any, for non-adherence. Clients should be asked to suggest what would make them more likely to adhere to medication, and this can be recorded on Worksheet 6 'Adherence to medication'.

> Many therapists have been trained to attribute non-adherence or failures in therapy to supposed personality characteristics or 'chronicity' of the client, rather than re-examining their own methods, their relationship with the client, or the meaning of the treatment for the client. Such a re-examination, together with a more equal treatment alliance, is likely to yield significant benefits to clients.
>
> *(Piatkowska and Farnhill, 1992)*

Experiences of using prescribed medication for schizophrenia

The National Schizophrenia Fellowship, MIND, and the Manic Depression Fellowship commissioned a large-scale research study to seek the views of people using medication for the treatment of severe mental illness. The results, based on 2,663 people, were published in two reports: 'A Question of Choice' (2000) and 'That's Just Typical' (2002). The latter focuses on people's experience of taking antipsychotic medication for schizophrenia. The findings, briefly outlined below, should be used to direct a discussion on clients experiences of medication, both good and bad.

- People prescribed 'typical' antipsychotics such as haloperidol, chlorpromazine and stelazine were less likely to be offered a choice of medication than those prescribed the newer 'atypical' antipsychotics such as clozapine, planzapine and risperidone.
- People prescribed typical antipsychotic agents were significantly more likely to have stopped taking their medication without the knowledge or support of their doctor (47 per cent). Over a third of those taking atypical agents had done the same (35 per cent). The main reason given for stopping their medication was the side effects.
- The most common side effects with typical antipsychotic agents were as follows: inner restlessness, 56 per cent; loss of energy, 53 per cent; muscle tremors, 48 per cent; weight gain, 46 per cent; muscle spasms, 40 per cent; effect on eyes, 38 per cent; sexual dysfunction, 35 per cent.
- The most common side effects with atypical antipsychotic agents were as follows: weight gain, 48 per cent; loss of energy, 33 per cent; inner restlessness, 23 per cent; sexual dysfunction, 20 per cent; effect on eyes, 18 per cent; muscle tremors, 13 per cent; muscle spasm, 6 per cent. Thus the newer medications seem to have considerably less negative effect than the older medications.

- The amount of information and involvement in the prescribing of medication was found to be rather poor. Only 50 per cent of patients were given any written information about possible side effects; 30 per cent were not involved in any discussion about their medication.
- While individuals experienced the effects of medication both positive and negative differently, there were some common opinions about medication. The survey asked: Which was the best medicine, and which was the worse medicine you have ever had? The top three were olanzapine $n = 175$; clozapine $n = 141$; risperidone $n = 107$. The worst: haloperidol $n = 344$; chlorpromazine $n = 256$; stelazine $n = 103$.

Assisting adherence to medication

The onus for improving adherence by ensuring good practice should be on ourselves as mental health professionals. In addition, the client's involvement and collaboration is vital. As a minimum, clients should be provided with the following:

1. Written information on the likely effects and side effects of their prescribed medication.
2. Informed choice of available medication options.
3. A regular medication review and the opportunity to discuss the effects and side effects with their prescriber.
4. A choice of trying a different medication if the first option is not acceptable.
5. Involvement in any decision to increase, decrease or change the medication.

Using medication notes as an aid, a retrospective review of previous medication, its effects and side effects should be constructed with the client. It can be helpful to plot known medication breaks and changes against the client's timeline to prompt recall of their personal medication history and effects of medication. Areas of exploration in order to improve adherence are presented below.

Checklist to explore improving adherence:

1. Knowledge – ensure that the client knows:
   - The purpose of the medication
   - The expected effects
   - The possible side effects
   - The expected time period for taking the medication
   - The right way to discontinue
   - Any drug interactions
   - When to take it and dosage.

2 Attitudes/beliefs
- Does the medication help the client?
- Do the benefits outweigh the costs?
- Does the client feel under pressure to take medication?
- Do they have any concerns about the medication?
- Do they think they are 'ill'/agree with their doctor?
- Do they have confidence in their doctor?
- What would happen if they stopped taking medication?

3 Subjective experience – explore how the client feels on the medication, eg

Drowsy	Tense
'Doped up'	Able to concentrate
More 'normal'	More sociable
More settled	Physically ill
Agitated	Think more clearly
Tired	Withdrawn
Relaxed	

Factors to consider in conducting a medication review with the client are presented in Box 11, and a formal assessment measure of attitude to medication, the Drug Attitude Inventory (Hogan et al, 1983), is also available.

> Each patient should ideally be prescribed only one antipsychotic, preferably in a single dosage form.
>
> *(Maudsley Prescribing Guidelines, 2001)*

Detailed recommendations for best practice in pharmacological interventions for schizophrenia are described in the National Institute for Clinical Excellence Clinical Guidelines (NICE, 2002). These include: first episode/early intervention medication; acute episode pharmacology including choice of antipsychotic; dosage and specific safeguards; post-acute and recovery phase medication.

BOX 11 Medication review

- Current experience of medication
  - positive effects
  - negative effects
  - subjective experience
- First experience of medication
  - positive and negative
- Periods of non-adherence
  - reasons for non-adherence
  - effects on mental health
- 'Drug free' trials (or 'drug holiday')
  - effects on mental health
- Changes in prescribed medication
  - reasons for changes
  - effects on mental health
  - polypharmacy effects
- Positive experience of medication
  - what do they find helpful and in what way
- Negative experience of medication
  - which medications did not suit them and in what way
- Effects of medication on other treatments
  - psychological interventions
  - effects on hospitalisation
- Physical health considerations
- Detailed dosage and drug regimen information if available

The problem-solving strategy (page 1 of 2)

There are seven steps to this strategy which will help you to become an effective problem solver.

Step 1: Define the problem

It is important to work out exactly what the problem is before attempting to solve it. A problem can be defined by asking where you are now and where you want to be, or what is the situation now and what do you want it to be. Try not to jump to solutions without fully understanding the problem.

Step 2: Stop and think

Thinking through problems before making decisions helps us to make better decisions. Taking all the information into account and reflecting on it stops us behaving impulsively.

Step 3: Gather information

To make good decisions it is important to have as much information as possible. The best sources of information are expert and independent.

Step 4: Generate alternatives

Try to think of several alternative solutions; you can use 'brainstorming' or ask other people for ideas.

Step 5: Think about the consequences

All decisions have 'pros' and 'cons'. It is important to consider all the costs and benefits before making a decision.

The problem-solving strategy (page 2 of 2)

Step 6: Planning

Before carrying out your decision, plan how to do this most effectively.

Step 7: Action

Do it!

Improving interpersonal performance (page 1 of 2)

Remember that what you say to yourself and how you feel will greatly influence your abilities to use your interpersonal skills. Controlling your emotions and thinking positively about your interactions will greatly improve your success in social situations.

Six successful strategies:

1 **Positive self-statements**

These are things you can say to yourself to make you feel better about yourself and your situation. Practise 'talking yourself up' with these statements, eg 'You are doing really well', 'You can do it', and 'You are good at this'.

2 **Thought switching**

Every time you catch yourself thinking negatively about yourself and your performance use this as a cue to switch to a more positive thought. You will have a number of pre-prepared positive self-statements; practise switching to these at every opportunity.

3 **Body language**

Research has shown that the actual words we use are responsible for only 7 per cent of the impact of the message. Our body language makes up 55 per cent of the impact and our voice – tone, speed volume – makes up the rest; it is often not what we say but how we say it that makes a difference. Practise your assertive stance, it will eventually feel natural!

Improving interpersonal performance (page 2 of 2)

An assertive stance consists of:

- Feet: hip width apart
- Legs: straight
- Hips: horizontal and not leaning
- Hands dropped in a relaxed manner
- Arms: shoulders back
- Head: raised and confident

4 Acting 'as if'

We all know how confident people would talk and behave in various situations. Even if you do not feel confident you can 'act confident'. This very simple strategy really works and soon becomes natural.

5 Covert relaxation

It is possible to go through physical relaxation strategies without anyone noticing. Pay particular attention to your shoulders and neck: drop your shoulders if they are raised, and tilt your head back slightly and relax your neck. You can go through each major muscle group, eg arms and legs, letting go of any tension.

6 Breathing and calming

Pay attention to your breathing, allowing it to become slow and steady. Calm yourself by imagining soothing words such as 'peace' and 'relax'.

Goal planning

Example (page 1 of 2)

Step 1: Establish the goals

Make a short list of what you would like to achieve in the next few months

Find better accommodation

Learn a skill to get a job

Earn some money

Get out more

Choose which one you would like to work on

'Get out more'

Step 2: Operationalise the goal

Specify the goal

I would like to do something regularly, which would get me out of the flat, and to which I could look forward.

Action plan

brainstorm all the things I could do

go to local library and find out what is available

choose one thing that I could try

do it!

Measure success

Make a list of what I have to do and tick off as it is achieved

Time allocated

Review in one month

Goal planning

Example (page 2 of 2)

Step 3: Carry out plan

Carry out your action plan, record or measure your progress

Brainstorm:

Exercise class, sport activity, dance class, yoga, interest groups, eg photography, walking, educational courses, eg natural history, astronomy, computers, assertiveness.

List for specific action plan	Tick when achieved
Brainstorm	✓
Telephone library and find out opening times	✓
Go to library	✓
Collect all available information on classes, courses and local groups	✓
Choose one activity	✓
Find out any further information needed, eg, telephone course leader	✓
Do it	✓

Step 4: Evaluate success

Review action plan and what you have achieved.

One month later have achieved everything on action plan. Joined local 'ramblers' walking group and have been on two walks already. Have met some nice people and look forward to next outing. Complete success!

Personal goal plan (page 1 of 2)

Step 1: Establish the goals

Make a short list of what you would like to achieve in the next few months

Choose which one you would like to work on

Step 2: Operationalise the goal

Specify the goal

Action plan

Measure success

Time allocated

Personal goal plan (page 2 of 2)

Step 3: Carry out plan

Carry out your action plan, record or measure your progress

List for specific action plan | Tick when achieved

Step 4: Evaluate success

Review action plan and what you have achieved.

Identification of stressors

(page 1 of 2)

Relationships with people – who?

- Family members
- Friends
- Professionals
- Workplace

Relationships with people – what?

Commonly, relationships are stressful because of the emotions they evoke and because of misunderstandings and 'communication' problems. People often find particular difficulty with relationships which they experience as: overprotective, controlling, critical, demanding, unsupportive, argumentative and overemotional.

Relationships with people – when?

The relationship is unlikely to always be stressful and you might find the relationship very positive most of the time. Commonly relationships have stress 'hot spots' at times when, eg the person's expectations of you do not match your own, there are financial problems, when personal habits cause annoyance to others.

Daily living problems

Our lives are complex and we routinely have to deal with people and situations which cause us stress. Even when there are no current problems associated with particular situations we have to 'keep on top' of them in order to prevent problems arising, eg pay bills, complete forms, answer correspondence.

Identification of stressors

(page 2 of 2)

Common sources of daily living stress include:

- Housing/accommodation
- Finances/money
- Work
- Social life/recreation
- Physical environment (eg comfort, noise, amenities)

Life events

It is well recognised that particular life events can cause significant stress and the more life events that are experienced in close proximity the harder they are to deal with effectively.

Common life events:

- Divorce or separation from partner
- Death of close friend or relative
- Change in employment
- Marriage
- Personal injury or illness
- Moving house or change in accommodation
- Imprisonment or arrest
- Injury or illness of close friend or relative
- Pregnancy and birth of child
- Significant change in financial circumstances

Internal stressors

In addition to stress from external sources we often put ourselves under stress by the way we think about ourselves and our interactions with other people.

Personal identification of stressors (page 1 of 3)

To use in conjunction with Handout 4 'Identification of stressors'

Relationships with people

Who, what and when

- Identify the particular relationships that sometimes cause you stress:

  ____

  ____

- Identify what it is about your experience of the relationship that causes most stress:

  ____

  ____

- Identify the types of situation that cause difficulty in these relationships:

  ____

  ____

Daily living problems

- Identify any current difficulties that you are experiencing in any of these areas:

  Housing/accommodation

  ____

  ____

  Finances

  ____

  ____

  Work

  ____

  ____

Personal identification of stressors (page 2 of 3)

Social life

Recreation

Physical environment

Life events

Have you experienced any of the following in the recent past (12 months)

- Divorce/separation from partner
- Death of close relative/friend
- Change in employment
- Marriage
- Personal injury or illness
- Move house or change in accommodation
- Imprisonment or arrest
- Injury or illness of close friend or relative
- Pregnancy and birth of child
- Significant change in financial circumstances
- Other significant life event

Personal identification of stressors (page 3 of 3)

Internal stressors

Identify the ways that you put yourself under pressure, eg

- Time urgency
- Being self-critical
- Being too concerned about my appearance
- Excessive worrying about minor problems
- Being too concerned about what other people think of me
- Trying to compete constantly with others
- Wanting approval/praise/attention from others
- Thinking the worst is going to happen
- Putting excessive demands on myself
- Other

Stress tracking example

Main stressors

Rate 0–10: 0 = stress not evident, 10 = stress extremely evident

1 Arguments with mother – monitor daily

Mon	Tue	Wed	Thu	Fri	Sat	Sun
10	*1*	*10*	*2*	*2*	*2*	*10*

2 Worrying about finances – monitor weekly

Week 1	Week 2	Week 3	Week 4	Week 5	Week 6	Week 7
6	*7*	*6*	*7*	*7*	*6*	*7*

3 Noisy neighbour – monitor daily

Mon	Tue	Wed	Thu	Fri	Sat	Sun
0	*0*	*0*	*10*	*10*	*10*	*0*

Stress signs and signals (page 1 of 2)

Our bodies, brains and behaviour can change in response to stress. We can use this to improve our awareness of stress by noticing 'early warning signs'. This provides us with a signal to take action to reduce the effects of stress.

Physical signs and signals

- Tiredness
- Increased susceptibility to colds, mouth ulcers, etc
- 'Butterflies' in stomach
- Nausea
- Palpitations
- Headaches and migraine
- Muscle tension
- Fast, shallow breathing
- Dizziness
- Diarrhoea
- Sweating
- Blushing

Psychological signs and signals

- Poor concentration
- Inability to make decisions
- Forgetfulness
- Disorganised/muddled thinking
- Negative thoughts
- Ruminating
- 'Obsessional' thinking
- Increase in thinking errors

Stress signs and signals (page 2 of 2)

Behavioural signs and signals

- Reduced performance
- Difficulty in clear communication
- Increased mistakes
- Aggression
- Crying
- Overactivity or underactivity
- Irritability
- Social withdrawal or avoidance
- Increased use of alcohol, cigarettes
- Overeating or undereating
- Clumsiness
- Insomnia
- Loss of sexual interest

My personal signs and signals of stress

Physical

Psychological

Behavioural

Strategies for coping with stress (page 1 of 2)

Healthy lifestyle

If you feel 'run down', tired or unhealthy it is much harder to deal with additional problems. Try to maintain your sense of well-being by:

- Making time for pleasurable activities
- Maintaining a healthy diet
- Exercising regularly, eg walking, swimming, exercise class, cycling
- Getting adequate sleep
- Prioritising relaxation

Support systems

Friends, relatives, colleagues and other supportive people can help to reduce the impact of stress in two contrasting ways: they can provide a distraction from your problems and they can help to make positive decisions and give a different perspective to problems: 'a problem shared is a problem halved'

Goal setting

Working out what you would like to achieve, how you are going to achieve your goals and evaluating your success will provide a sense of direction and control over your life

Problem solving

Some problems 'sort themselves out' but most do not! Identifying the problem, working out action plans and likely outcomes will help you to clarify your thoughts and make positive decisions

Strategies for coping with stress (page 2 of 2)

Prioritising

If you are feeling overwhelmed by problems it can seem as though you do not know where to start: start by prioritising! Deciding which problem or source of stress needs to be addressed most urgently can make the task more manageable. Sometimes it is easier to start with the most straightforward problems and build up to the more complex; once you have one success the next is more achievable.

Assertiveness

Clear and straightforward communication will help people to understand how you think and feel about a situation. Effective communication is often the best way to solve problems, or prevent them developing.

Challenge negative thinking

When under stress it is easy to slip into negative thinking styles such as catastrophising, expecting the worst, black-and-white thinking and personalising. Try to stay objective and examine problems in a realistic productive way.

Coping with stress record sheet: example

Source of stress	Stress rating (0–10)	My coping response	Stress rating afterwards (0–10)
Argument with friend	*6*	*Talked to mum about it*	*2*
Being self-critical ('beating myself up')	*8*	*Used cognitive coping strategy learnt in therapy session*	*1*
Computer course	*7*	*Talk to tutor about my difficulty*	*3*
Friend coming to visit	*9*	*Self-calming statements, relaxation*	*2*
Television not working	*5*	*Got TV repair man*	*0*
Flatmate untidiness	*10*	*Set up agreed rota for cleaning*	*2*

MODULE 4

Coping with stress record sheet

Source of stress	Stress rating (0–10)	My coping response	Stress rating afterwards (0–10)

Activity schedule: John

(page 1 of 4)

John is a 39-year-old man currently living in a group home. He has recently become quite withdrawn and spends most of his time sitting in the day room on his own. He rarely initiates conversation and is monosyllabic in his responses to questions.

1 He completed an *activity schedule* for one week; these are his first three days.

	Mon	Tue	Wed
9–10	*Breakfast*	*Breakfast*	*Breakfast*
10–11	*Sat in day room*	*Sat in day room*	*Sat in day room*
11–12	*Sat in day room*	*Sat in day room*	*Sat in day room*
12–1	*Lunch*	*Lunch*	*Lunch*
1–2	*Watched TV*	*Went for a walk*	*Read newspaper*
2–3	*Wrote a letter*	*Went to gardening*	*Went to gardening*
3–4	*Sat in day room*	*Sat in day room*	*Sat in day room*
4–5	*Made phone call*	*Listened to radio*	*Listened to radio*
5–6	*Supper*	*Supper*	*Supper*
6–7	*Had a bath*	*Listened to radio*	*Talked to EF*
7–8	*Watched TV*	*Tidied room*	*Did laundry*
8–9	*Watched TV*	*Watched TV*	*Watched TV*
9–10	*Watched TV*	*Watched TV*	*Watched TV*
10–11	*Went to bed*	*Went to bed*	*Went to bed*

Activity schedule: John

2 A review of the week's activity schedule found that John was more likely to engage in activities in the afternoon. He was also doing more than others thought he was.

3 Exploration of consequences of inactivity:
- Feel empty, alone, shut off
- Other people criticise me, tell me to do more
- Have given up reading, chess, drawing

4 Cognitive challenges

Elicited thoughts	*Exploration/challenges*
I can't cope with people	There are one or two people I get along with. Sometimes I like to talk to AB and CD
I can't concentrate on books anymore	Perhaps if I tried to read for 20 minutes each day I could build up my concentration
I have not got anyone to play chess with	Actually I have not asked anyone if they would like to play
What is the point of doing anything, it won't make me feel better	This is not necessarily true and it certainly can't make me feel worse

Activity schedule: John

(page 3 of 4)

5 Action plan to increase activity

Goal 1: to read a book

Steps:

1 Go to the library

2 Find a book by favourite author

3 Schedule in 20 minutes reading per day

Goal 2: to play a game of chess

Steps:

1 Ask AB/CD and/or EF if they would like a game of chess

2 Arrange a time for a game of chess

3 Set up board at appointed time and play

Goal 3: to rate activities for mastery and pleasure

6 Complete activity schedule for following week, using mastery and pleasure ratings and scheduling in new goal activities.

Activity schedule: John

(page 4 of 4)

	Mon	Tue	Wed
9–10	*Breakfast* *M2 P3*	*Breakfast* *M3 P3*	*Breakfast* *M3 P4*
10–11	*Sat in day room* *M2 P32*	*Sat in day room* *M2 P2*	*Sat in day room* *M2 P2*
11–12	*Listened to radio* *M3 P5*	*Sat in day room* *M2 P2*	*Sat in day room* *M2 P2*
12–1	*Lunch* *M4 P4*	*Lunch* *M4 P5*	*Lunch* *M4 P7*
1–2	*Watched TV* *M3 P4*	*Watched TV* *M3 P4*	*Read 20 mins* *M6 P7*
2–3	*Sat in day room* *M2 P2*	*Watched TV* *M3 P4*	*Listened to radio* *M4 P6*
3–4	*Sat in day room* *M2 P2*	*Watched TV* *M3 P4*	*Listened to radio* *M4 P6*
4–5	*To library* *M7 P7*	*Listened to radio* *M5 P6*	*Listened to radio* *M5 P7*
5–6	*Supper* *M4 P6*	*Supper* *M4 P6*	*Supper* *M4 P6*
6–7	*Read 20 mins* *M5 P6*	*Played chess* *M8 P9*	*Played chess* *M8 P9*
7–8	*Bath* *M5 P6*	*TV* *M5 P6*	*Bath* *M5 P6*
8–9	*TV* *M3 P4*	*TV* *M4 P7*	*TV* *M4 P6*
9–10	*TV/bed* *M3 P4*	*TV/bed* *M3 P6*	*TV/bed* *M3 P4*
10–11			

Pleasurable activities

Sporting event, eg football match

Read a book

Watch TV

Meet a friend

Relax in a warm bath

Listen to music

Go to cinema

Play games, for example pool, darts, cards, chess

Spend time with pets

Cook a meal

Go for a walk

Have a picnic

Go horse riding

Go fishing

Gardening

Go to the library

Social event

Go on a day trip

Get a takeaway meal

Go out for a meal

Pampering: hairdressers, manicure, etc

Shopping

Play sport/other activity, eg swimming

Play music

Go to a concert, theatre

Go to the park, countryside

DIY

Art, craft

Collecting, eg stamps, fossils

Activity schedule

	Mon	Tue	Wed	Thu	Fri	Sat	Sun
9–10							
10–11							
11–12							
12–1							
1–2							
2–3							
3–4							
4–5							
5–6							
6–7							
7–8							
8–9							
9–10							
10–11							

Reasons for non-adherence

- Subjective experience of the medication
  This is how you feel on the medication, subjective experience can be positive, eg feeling more like your usual self, or negative, eg feeling tired and sluggish.
- Health beliefs
  If you believe that medication might make you ill, or that you do not need medication because you are not ill this is likely to affect adherence.
- Attitude to medication
  You might think that you do not need to take medication once you feel better; this is not the case with 'maintenance' medication which can help to prevent a relapse.
- Relationship with prescriber
  Having trust in your doctor and being able to talk openly and honestly about the medication and its effects will help you to feel more confident in the medication prescribed.
- Beliefs of family/friends
  If your family/friends are supportive and accepting of your problems and understand the benefits of medication this is likely to influence your use of medication.
- Medication side effects
  Sometimes medication can produce unpleasant side effects, such as feeling very tired, weight gain and shakiness. If these symptoms are being caused by the medication it might be helpful to alter the dose of medication or perhaps take additional medication specifically to reduce the side effects.

MODULE 4

Adherence to medication

I would be more likely to adhere to my medication if ...

Bringing it all together

MODULE 5

Overview of Module

- Introduction
- Evaluation of progress
- Review of monitoring forms
- Review of aims and goals
- Review of phases of schizophrenia
- Review of protective factors
- Future directions

Suggested Session Plans

Individual completion of psychometric assessments and feedback	**45 min**
Individual interview to assess changes and feedback	**45 min**
Evaluation of progress	**10 min**
General feedback from assessments	**15 min**
Review of monitoring forms	**20 min**
Review of personal aims	**15 min**
Review of goal planning	**15 min**
Review of longer-term goals	**15 min**

Review of phases of schizophrenia and compilation of relapse recognition and action plans	**40 min**
Review of interpersonal effectiveness strategies and revision of hierarchies	**20 min**
Review of stress management	**20 min**
Complete programme evaluation form	**10 min**
Identifying unmet needs	**20 min**
Local and national resources	**20 min**
Question and answer session	**20 min**
Tea and cakes and certificates!	**30 min**

Introduction

This module has two main aims. First, to review and consolidate what has been learnt throughout the programme, and second, to examine future plans and directions.

Evaluation of progress

Change in clients can be formally evaluated by using psychometric questionnaires. Repeating the measures that clients completed prior to the intervention, will illustrate any progress. The questionnaires might include assessments of symptomatology such as the Comprehensive Psychopathological Rating Scale (CPRS); depression, eg Beck Depression Inventory (BDI); interpersonal problems, eg Inventory of Interpersonal Problems (IIP 32); social anxiety, eg Fear of Negative Evaluation (FNE), Social Avoidance and Distress scale (SAD) and self-esteem, eg Self-Concept Questionnaire (SCQ). The results of any 'before' and 'after' measures should be discussed with the clients in order to illustrate those areas in which positive changes have occurred. The feedback should be given on an individual basis.

A simple and effective way of evaluating change and illustrating progress to clients is to repeat a series of questions that the clients were asked prior to the interventions. This again should be conducted on a one-to-one basis, and feedback of changes discussed with clients. Example questions might include:

- Do you think that you have a mental health problem?
- Do you think that mental health services can help you in any way?
- How do you explain your ...? (unusual beliefs/voices/other phenomena)
- Do you have some ideas about how to manage your mental health problems?
- Do you notice any change in your symptoms over time?
- Does anything make the symptoms worse/better?
- Can you recognise when you are becoming mentally unwell?

Comparing clients' answers with those given before interventions can highlight improvements in knowledge, awareness and self-efficacy.

Review of monitoring forms

Review all monitoring forms and personal questionnaires which clients have kept over the course of the programme. These will have been reviewed perhaps weekly for specific purposes, such as monitoring hallucinations in order to identify precipitants and to monitor changes in delusional experiences. However, a complete review of such self-monitoring can provide useful information to illustrate reductions in distress ratings, improved coping strategies and increased self-awareness. Include the following monitoring worksheets in the review:

- Hallucination monitoring record (Part III, Module 3, Worksheet 1)
- Diary sheet for monitoring symptoms (Part III, Module 3, Worksheet 2)
- Coping with stress record sheet (Part III, Module 4, Handout 8)
- Activity schedule (Part III, Module 4, Worksheet 5).

Also review Module 4 'Stress tracking', Module 3 'Personal questionnaires' and any personal diary work.

Review of aims and goals

Remind clients of their personal aims that they set at the beginning of the programme. Refer to Module 1 Worksheet 2 'My personal aims', in which clients recorded what they would like to get out of participating in the programme, which might have included specific learning objectives, specific areas for improvement and potential achievements. Ask each group member to what extent their aims have been achieved, and explore ways of meeting any aims which were not fully realised.

Clients should be referred to Module 4 Worksheet 1 'Personal goal plan', in which they listed a number of short-term goals which they would like to achieve, and the steps to follow in goal planning. Invite clients to add to or modify any of their goals. Remind clients that goal planning is an ongoing process and that they should continue to work at achieving their goals.

Clients should be referred to Module 2 Worksheet 8 'Future me', in which they identified goals for the next year. Discuss these in terms of their current relevance, priority and how to achieve them.

Review of phases of schizophrenia

Module 2 enabled clients to examine their personal experiences of the onset and course of their symptoms. This can be reviewed to remind clients of salient information and how this can be used, both to signal potential relapse and to communicate effectively about their symptoms. Module 3 provided coping strategies and improved self-efficacy in managing symptoms.

Collate the following worksheets from Module 2:

- Worksheet 3, 'Identification of prodromal signs';
- Worksheet 4, 'Responses to prodromal signs';
- Worksheet 5, 'My acute phase';
- Worksheet 6, 'My recovery phase';
- Worksheet 7, 'Early warning signs action plan'.

From Module 3, collate the following:

- Worksheet 2, 'Diary sheet for monitoring symptoms';
- Worksheet 3, 'Objective examination of belief',
- Worksheet 4, 'Behavioural experiment'.

Help clients to use the information gathered to assemble a comprehensive relapse recognition and action plan, and to complete Module 5, Worksheet 1 'Relapse Recognition and Action Plan'. As well as salient information from their worksheets, include any supplementary information or detail to make the plan as clear and as useful as possible.

Review of protective factors

Remind the group of the protective factors covered during Module 4.

Review interpersonal effectiveness sessions by reminding the group of the problem-solving steps and ask for examples in which clients had used problem solving either successfully or unsuccessfully. Further role play and discussion sessions should be undertaken as appropriate. Remind the group of the specific skills practised, for example asking for help, apologising, convincing others, assertiveness, negotiation and the role of emotion and cognition in affecting our performance.

Refer clients to the hierarchies they constructed of difficult social situations and review their progress. Hierarchies can be revised as necessary. Remind clients that this work is ongoing and that every social situation is an opportunity to practise and consolidate their skills. Similarly, encourage those with inactivity, motivation and social withdrawal difficulties to continue with their activity schedules and mastery and pleasure ratings, also review their graded exposure hierarchies and modify as appropriate.

Review interventions for stress. Refer clients to the following records from Module 4: Worksheet 2 'Personal identification of stressors'; Worksheet 3 'My personal signs and signals of stress'; and Worksheet 4 'Coping with stress record sheet'. Ask clients to prepare a short – five-minute – talk on what they have learnt about their personal stressors and how to identify and cope with them. They should then present this to the group.

At the end of this session, ask clients to evaluate the programme and its impact on them; an evaluation sheet is provided in Module 5, Worksheet 2 'Programme evaluation form'.

Future directions

During the review sessions, areas of continuing or unmet needs might have been identified. The collaborative approach is likely to identify needs which the client themselves would like to address. Helping clients to express and work on their own areas of need should be comparative, that is, based on the position of other individuals or reference groups, such as other group members, rather than on the judgement and values of professionals (Bradshaw, 1972).

A more formal process for assessing the needs for treatment and care is the Medical Research Council (MRC) 'Needs for Care Assessment' (Brewin et al, 1987). This covers 21 areas of clinical and social functioning, and for each specifies appropriate interventions. It classifies each need as either met, unmet or no need. The areas of functioning are divided into symptoms and behavioural problems, such as positive symptoms, side effects of medication and physical disorder, and into personal and social skills such as management of money, occupational skills and social interaction skills. This can be a useful reference to ensure that no areas of need have been missed.

Spend sufficient time addressing any further areas of need that clients would like to work on, and ensuring the best ways of achieving this. This might include continuing individual sessions with their therapist or referral to other professionals or agencies. A 'maintenance' group for clients should be offered, if at all possible. This allows the group members to meet regularly but less frequently, for example once a month. The maintenance group serves to consolidate learning, practise skills, rehearse strategies and so on, as well as enabling group members to retain contact with each other and with the facilitators.

It is very helpful to compile a brochure of what is available for clients locally with information about how to access services. This might include the following.

- List of mental health professionals. Give the name and contact details for each professional, for example psychologist, psychiatrist, care coordinator, social worker, occupational therapist, general practitioner, assertive outreach team contact and emergency contact.
- Contact details of all useful services including general hospital, psychiatric hospital, day centre, hostels, social services, housing and accommodation, local employment office.
- Contact details for community facilities such as local social activities, recreation/leisure centres, education establishments, libraries.
- Contact details of all local voluntary organisations, for example user and carer groups, self-help support groups and any local branches of national organisations such as MIND and Rethink.

Information on national organisations is provided in Handout 1 'Useful links and organisations'.

The last session should be less formal and tea and cakes could be provided. Allow each group member and facilitator the opportunity to tell the group their thoughts about participating in the programme and the ending of the group. Thank everyone for their participation. Provide group members with a signed, and if possible laminated certificate of attendance.

Relapse recognition and action plan (page 1 of 2)

My prodromal signs are:

My usual responses to each sign are:

My acute phase symptoms and responses are:

What makes my symptoms worse:

(ignoring them, stress, other precipitants)

Relapse recognition and action plan (page 2 of 2)

What can make my symptoms better:

(eg list coping strategies, objective examination, challenges)

My most useful medication and dosage is:

My action plan:

(outline your action plan for responding to early warning signs/symptoms, including detail of timescales, telephone numbers, etc)

Programme evaluation form

What did you like most about the programme?

____

____

What did you like least about the programme?

____

____

How would you improve the programme?

____

____

Please rate on a 1–5 scale: 1 = not at all; 5 = greatly, to what extent participation in the programme:

- Increased your knowledge of schizophrenia ____
- Increased your understanding of yourself and your mental health ____
- Helped you to cope more effectively with mental health problems ____
- Helped you to improve your skills at dealing with other people ____
- Helped you to feel better about yourself and your situation ____
- To what extent did the programme meet your personal aims? ____

Any other comments

____

____

____

Thank you

Useful links and organisations

(page 1 of 5)

Mental health organisations in the UK

Rethink (previously National Schizophrenia Fellowship)

Provides information on types of mental illness and treatments, living with severe mental health difficulties, money and benefits, legal matters, information and advice.

Rethink
Head Office
30 Tabernacle Street
LONDON EC2A 4DD
Tel: 0845 456 0455
www.rethink.org

Rethink
28 Castle Street
KINGSTON-UPON-THAMES
Surrey KT1 1SS
Tel: 0845 456 0455
email: info@rethink.org

National Advice Service

Staffed by advisers with knowledge about severe mental health problems.

Tel: 020 8974 6814 (10.00 am–3.00 pm, Monday to Friday)
email: advice@rethink.org

The National Schizophrenia Fellowship of Scotland

Information and services for people with mental illness and their carers living in Scotland.

www.nsfscot.org.uk

Carers UK

A large national charity working on behalf of carers.

www.carers.org.uk

Useful links and organisations

(page 2 of 5)

The Manic Depression Fellowship

Information about bipolar disorder.

www.mdf.org.uk

The Mental Health Foundation

Information about mental health, rights and about the Foundation.

www.mentalhealth.org.uk

Emotional Support Network

Offers a support network around the UK for people in need of emotional support.

www.emotionalsupport.net

The Sainsbury Centre for Mental Health

Information about projects run by the Centre to improve mental health services.

www.scmh.org.uk

SANE

SANE is a national charity working to improve the quality of life for people affected by mental health problems.

SANELINE 0845 767 8000 (12 noon–2.00 am, daily)

Helpline for information and support.

www.sane.org.uk

Useful links and organisations

(page 3 of 5)

Money and benefits

Benefit Enquiry Line

General information about benefits for people with disabilities and their carers.

Tel: 0800 882200

Disability Benefit Customer Care Helpline

For claimants with an enquiry on their disability living allowance or attendance claim.

Tel: 0845 712 3456

The Department for Work and Pensions

Government information on benefits, pensions and work-related issues.

www.dwp.gov.uk

Job Centre Plus

Provides information on benefits for people of working age, information on employment and schemes for getting into work.

www.jobcentreplus.gov.uk

National Debtline

Advice about mortgage and rent arrears and other debt.

Tel: 0808 808 4000

www.nationaldebtline.co.uk

Useful links and organisations

Work and education

Skill: The National Bureau for Students with Disabilities

Provides information and advice about opportunities in post-16 education, training and employment.

www.skill.org.uk

The National Centre for Volunteering

Database of local organisations looking for volunteers.

www.volunteering.org.uk

First Step Trust

Runs projects providing services such as decorating, gardening and office administration. The projects are run and staffed by people with mental health problems, drug or alcohol problems or learning difficulties.

www.fst.org.uk

Useful links and organisations

(page 5 of 5)

Healthcare

National Health Service

The NHS website has information about the NHS and its services.

www.nhs.uk

NHS Direct

Provides a 24-hour health information service in the UK.

www.nhsdirect.org.uk

Web4Health

An organisation sponsored by the European Commission. Site contains free medical advice on mental health, psychology, relationships, stress, etc.

www.web4health.info

Bibliography

American Psychiatric Association, 2000, *Diagnostic and Statistical Manual of Mental Disorders*, 4th edn, Text Revision (DSM-IV-TR).

Ananth J & Ghadirian AM, 1980, 'Drug Induced Mood Disorder', *International Pharmacopsychiatry* 15, pp58–73.

Andreasen NC, 1981, *The Scale For The Assessment of Negative Symptoms SANS*, University of Iowa, Iowa City, Iowa.

Andreasen NC, 1984, *Scale for the Assessment of Positive Symptoms SAPS*, Department of Psychiatry, University of Iowa, Iowa City, Iowa.

Asberg M, Montgomery S, Perris C, Schalling D & Sedvall G, 1978, 'The Comprehensive Psychopathological Rating Scale', *Acta Psychiatrica Scandinavica* Supplement 271, pp5–27.

Babiker IE, 1986, 'Non-compliance in Schizophrenia', *Psychiatry Dev* 4, pp329–37.

Bandura A, 1977, 'Self-Efficacy: Toward a Unifying Theory of Behavioural Change', *Psychological Review* 84, pp191–215.

Barkham M, Hardy GE & Startup M, 1996, 'The IIP-32: A Short Version of the Inventory of Interpersonal Problems', *British Journal of Clinical Psychology* 35, pp21–35.

Barnes TRE & Nelson HE, 1994, *The Assessment of Psychoses: A Practical Handbook*, Chapman & Hall Medical, London.

Barofsky I & Connelly CE, 1983, 'Problems in Providing Effective Care for the Chronic Psychiatric Patient' in I Barofsy & RO Budson (eds), *The Chronic Psychiatric Patient in the Community: Principles of Treatment*, SP Medical and Scientific, New York, pp83–119.

Beck AT, 1994, 'Foreword', in DG Kingdon & D Turkington (eds), *Cognitive-behavioural Therapy of Schizophrenia*, Guildford Press, New York.

Beck AT, Rush AJ, Shaw BF & Emery G, 1979, *Cognitive Therapy of Depression*, Guildford Press, New York.

Beck AT, Ward CH, Mendelson M, Mock JE & Erbaugh JK, 1961, 'An Inventory for Measuring Depression', *Comprehensive Psychiatry Journal* 2, pp163–70.

Bentall R, Haddock G & Slade P, 1994, 'Cognitive Behaviour Therapy for Persistent Auditory Hallucinations: From Theory to Therapy', *Behaviour Therapy* 25, pp51–66.

Bentall RP, 1990, *Reconstructing Schizophrenia*, Routledge, London.

Benton MK & Schroeder HE, 1990, 'Social Skills Training with Schizophrenics: A Meta-Analytic Evaluation', *Journal of Consulting and Clinical Psychology* 58, pp741–7.

Birchwood MJ, Hallet SE & Preston MC, 1988, *Schizophrenia: An Integrated Approach to Research and Treatment*, Longman, London.

Birchwood M, Smith J, MacMillan F, Hogg B, Prasad R, Harvey C & Bering S, 1989, 'Predicting Relapse in Schizophrenia: The Development and Implementation of an Early Signs Monitoring System Using Patients and Families as Observers, A Preliminary Investigation', *Psychological Medicine* 19, pp649–56.

Birchwood M, MacMillan F & Smith J, 1992, *Early Intervention'*, in M Birchwood & N Tarrier (eds), *Innovations in the Psychological Management of Schizophrenia,* John Wiley & Sons Ltd, Chichester.

Bradshaw, J, 1972, 'A Taxonomy of Social Need', G McLachlan (ed), in *Problems and Progress in Medical Care,* Seventh Series, OUP, London, pp71–82.

Breier A & Strauss JS, 1983, 'Self-Control in Psychotic Disorders', *Archives of General Psychiatry* 40, pp1141–5.

Brett-Jones J, Garety P & Hemsley D, 1987, 'Measuring Delusional Experiences: A Method and its Application', *British Journal of Clinical Psychology* 26, pp257–65.

Brewin CR, Wing JK & Mangen TS, 1987, 'Principles and Practice of Measuring Needs in the Long-Term Mentally Ill: The MRC Needs for Care Assessment', *Psychological Medicine* 17, pp971–81.

British Psychological Society, 2000, 'Understanding Mental Illness. Recent Advances in Understanding Mental Illness and Psychotic Experiences', Report by BPS Division of Clinical Psychology.

Brown GW, Birley JLT & Wing JK, 1972, 'Influence of Family Life on the Course of Schizophrenic Disorders; Replication', *British Journal of Psychiatry*, 121, pp241–58.

Carr V, 1988, 'Patients' Techniques for Coping with Schizophrenia: An Exploratory Study', *British Journal of Medical Psychology*, 61 pp339–52.

Chadwick P & Birchwood M, 1994, 'The Omnipotence of Voices: A Cognitive Approach to Auditory Hallucinations', *British Journal of Psychiatry* 164 pp190–201.

Chadwick P & Birchwood M, 1995, 'The Omnipotence of Voices II: the Beliefs About Voices Questionnaire BAVQ', *British Journal of Psychiatry* 166 pp773–6.

Chadwick P & Lowe CF, 1990, 'The Measurement and Modification of Delusional Beliefs', *Journal of Consulting and Clinical Psychology* 58, pp225–32.

Chadwick P & Lowe CF, 1994, 'A Cognitive Approach to Measuring and Modifying Delusions', *Behaviour Research and Therapy* 32, pp355–67.

Claridge G, 1990, 'Can a Disease Model of Schizophrenia Survive?', in RP Bentall (ed), *Reconstructing Schizophrenia*, Routledge, London.

Cohen CI & Berk LA, 1985, 'Personal Coping Styles of Schizophrenic Outpatients', *Hospital and Community Psychiatry* 36, pp407–10.

Curson DA, Barnes TRE & Bamber RW, 1985, 'Long-term Depot Maintenance of Chronic Schizophrenic Outpatients', *British Journal of Psychiatry* 146, pp464–80.

Curson DA, Patel M & Liddle PF, 1988, 'Psychiatric Morbidity of a Long-stay Hospital Population with Chronic Schizophrenia and Implications for Future Community Care', *British Medical Journal* 297, pp811–22.

David AS, 1990, 'Insight and Psychosis', *British Journal of Psychiatry* 156, pp798–808.

Drury V, Birchwood M, Cochrane R et al, 1996, 'Cognitive Therapy and Recovery from Acute Psychosis: A Controlled Trial 1 Impact on Psychotic Symptoms', *British Journal of Psychiatry* 169, pp593–601.

Eckman TA & Liberman RP, 1990, 'A Large-scale Field Test of a Medication Management Skills Training Program for People with Schizophrenia', *Psychosocial Rehabilitation Journal* 13 (3), pp31–35.

Emmelkamp PMG, 1994, 'Behaviour therapy with Adults', in AE Bergin & SL Garfield (eds), *Handbook of Psychotherapy and Behaviour Change,* 4th edn, Wiley, New York.

Falloon I, Watt DC & Shepherd M, 1978, 'A Comparative Controlled Trial of Pimozide and Fluphenazine Diaconate in the Continuation Therapy of Schizophrenia', *Psychological Medicine* 8, pp59–70.

Falloon IRH, Boyd JL, McGill CW, Ranzini J, Moss HB & Gilderman AM, 1982, 'Family Management in the Prevention of Exacerbation in Schizophrenia: A Controlled Study', *New England Journal of Medicine* 306, pp1437–40.

Falloon IRH & Talbot RE, 1981, 'Persistent Auditory Hallucinations: Coping Mechanisms and Implications for Management', *Psychological Medicine* 11, pp329–39.

Garety PA 1985, 'Delusions: Problems in Definition and Measurement', *British Journal of Medical Psychology* 58, pp25–34.

Garety PA, Kuipers L, Fowler D, Chamberlain F & Dunn G, 1994, 'Cognitive Behaviour Therapy for Drug Resistant Psychosis', *British Journal of Medical Psychology* 67, pp259–71.

Gilbert PC, Harris J, McAdams LA & Jeste DV, 1995, 'Neuroleptic Withdrawal in Schizophrenic Patients: A Review of the Literature', *Archives of General Psychiatry* 52, pp173–88.

Gregory RL, 1979, *Eye and Brain: The Psychology of Seeing*, Weidenfeld & Nicholson, London.

Goldstein AP, 1999, *The Prepare Curriculum: Teaching Prosocial Competencies*, Research Press, Illinois.

Haddock G, Tarrier N, Spaulding W, Yusupoff L, Kinney C & McCarthy E, 1998, 'Individual Cognitive Behaviour Therapy in the Treatment of Hallucinations and Delusions: A Review', *Clinical Psychology Review* 18, pp821–38.

Hamilton M, 1960, 'A Rating Scale for Depression', *Journal of Neurology, Neurosurgery and Psychiatry* 23, pp56–62.

Herz MI & Melville C, 1980, 'Relapse in Schizophrenia', *American Journal of Psychiatry* 137, pp801–5.

Hogan TP, Awad AG & Eastwood R, 1983, 'A Self-report Scale Predictive of Drug Compliance in Schizophrenics: Reliability and Discriminative Validity', *Psychological Medicine* 13, pp177–83.

Hogarty GE, 1984, 'Depot Neuroleptic: The Relevance of Psychosocial Factors', *Journal of Clinical Psychiatry* 2, pp36–42.

Horowitz LM, Rosenberg SE, Baer BA, Vreno G & Villasenor VS, 1988, 'Inventory of Interpersonal Problems, Psychometric Properties and Clinical Applications', *Journal of Consulting and Clinical Psychology* 56, pp885–92.

Johnson DAW, 1993, 'Depot Neuroleptics, in TRF Barnes (ed), *Antipsychotic Drugs and their Side-effects'*, Academic Press, London, pp205–12.

Johnstone E, 1989, 'The Assessment of Positive and Negative Features in Schizophrenia', *British Journal of Psychiatry* 155 (Suppl 7), pp41–4.

Kay SR, Opler LA & Lindenmayer JP, 1989, 'The Positive and Negative Syndrome Scale PANSS: Rationale and Standardisation', *British Journal of Psychiatry* 155 (Suppl 7), pp59–65.

Kingdon DG & Turkington D, 1994, *Cognitive-behavioural Therapy for Schizophrenia*, Erlbaum, Hove.

Krawiecka M, Goldberg D & Vaughan M, 1977, 'A Standardised Psychiatric Assessment Scale for Rating Chronic Psychiatric Patients', *Acta Psychiatricia Scandinavica* 55 pp299–308.

Kuipers E, Garety PA, Fowler D, Dunn G, Bebbington P, Freeman D & Hadley D, 1997, 'London – East Anglia Randomised Controlled Trial of Cognitive-behavioural Therapy for Psychosis 1: Effects of Treatment Phase', *British Journal of Psychiatry* 171, pp 319–27.

Kuipers E & Moore E, 1995, 'Expressed Emotion and Staff Client Relationships: Implications for the Community Care of the Severely Mental Ill', *International Journal of Mental Health* 24, pp13–26.

Lam DH, 1991, 'Psychosocial Family Intervention in Schizophrenia: A Review of Empirical Studies', *Psychological Medicine* 21, pp423–41.

Liddle PF & Barnes TRE, 1988, 'The Subjective Experience of Deficits in Schizophrenia', *Comprehensive Psychiatry* 29, pp157–64.

Lindsay PH & Norman DA, 1977, *Human Information Processing*, Academic Press, London.

MacMillan JF, Crow TJ, Johnson AL & Johnstone EC, 1986, 'The Northwick Park First Episodes of Schizophrenia Study', *British Journal of Psychiatry* 148, pp128–33.

McEvoy JP, Apperson LJ, Appelbaum PS, Ortlip P, Brecosky J, Hammill K, Geller JL & Roth L, 1989, 'Insight in Schizophrenia: Its Relationship to Acute Psychopathology', *Journal of Nervous and Mental Disease* 177, pp43–7.

McEvoy JP, Freter S, Everett G et al, 1989b, 'Insight and the Clinical Outcome of Schizophrenic Patients', *Journal of Nervous and Mental Disease* 177 pp48–51.

Marder SR, Mebane A, Chien CP, Winslade WJ, Swann E & Van Putten T, 1983, 'A Comparison of Patients who Refuse and Consent to Neuroleptic Treatment', *American Journal of Psychiatry* 140, pp470–2.

Margo A, Hemsley DR & Slade P, 1981, 'The Effects of Varying Auditory Input on Schizophrenic Hallucinations', *British Journal of Psychiatry* 139, pp122–7.

Marlatt GA & Gordon JR, 1985, *Relapse Prevention: Maintenance Strategies in the Treatment of Addictive Behaviours*, Guildford Press, New York.

Morrison AP & Haddock G, 1997, 'Cognitive Factors in Source Monitoring and Auditory Hallucinations', *Psychological Medicine* 27, pp669–79.

National Institute for Clinical Excellence (NICE), 2002, *Clinical Guideline One. Schizophrenia. Core Interventions in the Treatment and Management of Schizophrenia in Primary and Secondary Care*, December.

Neuchterlein KH, 1987, 'Vulnerability models for Schizophrenia: State of the Art', in H Hafner, WF Gattaz & W Janzarik (eds), *Search for the Causes of Schizophrenia*, Springer-Verlag, Heidelberg, pp297–316.

Nuechterlein KH & Dawson ME, 1984, 'A Heuristic Vulnerability–Stress Model of Schizophrenic Episodes', *Schizophrenia Bulletin* 10, pp300–12.

Nyani TH & David AS, 1996, 'The Auditory Hallucination: A Phenomendogical Survey', *Psychological Medicine* 26, pp177–89.

Overall JE & Gorham DR, 1962, 'The Brief Psychiatric Rating Scale', *Psychological Reports* 10, pp799–812.

Piatkowska OE & Farnill D, 1992, 'Medication – compliance or Alliance? A Client-centred Approach to Increasing Adherence', in DJ Kavanagh (ed), *Schizophrenia: An Overview and Practical Handbook*, Chapman and Hall, London, pp339–55.

Padesky C, 1993, 'Schema as Self-prejudice', *International Cognitive Therapy Newsletter* 5/6, pp16–17.

Prochaska JO & Di Clemente CC, 1982, 'Transtheoretical Therapy: Towards a More Integrative Model of Change', *Psychotherapy: Theory Research and Practice* 19 (3).

Prosser ES, Csernansky JG, Kaplan J, Thiemann S, Becker TJ & Hollister LE, 1987, 'Depression Parkinsonian Symptoms and Negative Symptoms in Schizophrenics Treated with Neuroleptics', *Journal of Nervous and Mental Disease* 175, pp100–5.

Robson P, 1989, 'Development of a New Self-report Questionnaire to Measure Self-esteem', *Psychological Medicine* 19, pp513–18.

Roth A & Fonagy P, 1996, *What Works for Whom? A Critical Review of Psychotherapy Research*, Guildford Press, New York.

Sackett DL & Haynes RB, 1976, *Compliance with Therapeutic Regimens*, Johns Hopkins University Press, Baltimore.

Shapiro MB, 1961, 'A Method of Measuring Psychological Disorders Specific to the Individual Psychiatric Patients', *British Journal of Medical Psychology* 34, pp151–5.

Shepherd M, Watt D, Falloon I & Smeeton N, 1989, 'The Natural History of Schizophrenia: A Five-year Follow-up of Outcome and Prediction in a Representative Sample of Schizophrenics', *Psychological Medicine Monograph* 16, Cambridge University Press, Cambridge.

Shergill SS, Murray RM & McGuire PK, 1998, 'Auditory Hallucinations: A Review of Psychological Treatments', *Schizophrenia Research* 32, pp137–50.

Slade PD, 1971, 'The Effects of Systematic Desensitisation on Auditory Hallucinations', *Behaviour Research and Therapy* 10, pp85–91.

Startup M, 1998, 'Insight and Interpersonal Problems in Long-term Schizophrenia', *Journal of Mental Health* 7 (3), pp299–308.

Tarrier N, 1992, 'Management and Modification of Residual Positive Psychotic Symptoms', in M Birchwood & N Tarrier (eds), *Innovations in the Psychological Management of Schizophrenia,* John Wiley and Sons Ltd, Chichester.

Torrey DF, 1987, 'Prevalence Studies of Schizophrenia', *British Journal of Psychiatry* 150, pp598–608.

Turkington D, John CH & Siddle R, 1996, 'Cognitive Therapy in the Treatment of Drug-resistant Delusional Disorder', *Clinical Psychology and Psychotherapy* 3, pp118–28.

Vaccaro JV & Roberts L, 1992, 'Teaching social and coping skills', in M Birchwood & N Tarrier (eds), *Innovations in the Psychological Management of Schizophrenia*, John Wiley and Sons Ltd, Chichester.

Vaughn CE & Leff JP, 1976, 'The Influence of Family and Social Factors on the Course of Psychiatric Illness', *British Journal of Psychiatry* 129, pp125–37.

Wallace CJ & Liberman RP, 1985, 'Social Skills Training for Schizophrenics: A Controlled Clinical Trial', *Psychiatry Research* 15, pp239–47.

Watson D & Friend R, 1969, 'Measurement of Social-evaluative Anxiety', *Journal of Consulting and Clinical Psychology* 33 (4), pp448–57.

Wing JK, Cooper JE & Sartorius N, 1974, *The Measurement and Classification of Psychiatric Symptoms*, Cambridge University Press, Cambridge.

World Health Organization, 1992, *ICD-10 Classification of Mental and Behavioural Disorders: Clinical Descriptions and Diagnostic Guidelines*, WHO, Geneva.

World Health Organization, 1973, *Report on the International Pilot Study of Schizophrenia*, WHO, Geneva.

Wright EC, 1993, 'Non-compliance – or How Many Aunts Has Matilda?', *The Lancet* 342, pp909–13.

Wykes T & Sturt E, 1986, 'The Measurement of Social Behaviour in Psychiatric Patients: An Assessment of the Reliability and Validity of the SBS Schedule', *British Journal of Psychiatry* 148, pp1–11.

Young J, 1991, *Cognitive Therapy for Personality Disorders*, Professional Resource Exchange, Sarasota, Florida.

Zubin J & Spring B, 1977, 'Vulnerability: A New View of Schizophrenia', *Journal of Abnormal Psychology* 86, pp260–6.